About the Author

Pixie Turner is a registered nutritionist and psychotherapist, and director of The Food Therapy Centre, where she specialises in emotional eating, eating disorders and body image. She is the author of four previous books: *The Wellness Rebel*, *Pixie's Plates*, *The No-Need-to-Diet Book* and *The Insta-Food Diet*. In 2020–21, she co-hosted (alongside cardiothoracic surgeon Nikki Stamp) *In Bad Taste*, a podcast that casts a critical eye over the content and claims of health documentaries.

Food Therapy

Understand and repair your
relationship with what you eat

Pixie Turner

PIATKUS

PIATKUS

First published in Great Britain in 2023 by Piatkus

1 3 5 7 9 10 8 6 4 2

A CIP catalogue record for this book
is available from the British Library.

ISBN 978-0-349-42931-1

Typeset in Calluna by M Rules
Printed and bound in Great Britain by
Clays Ltd, Elcograf S.p.A

Papers used by Piatkus are from well-managed forests
and other responsible sources.

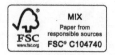

Piatkus
An imprint of
Little, Brown Book Group
Carmelite House
50 Victoria Embankment
London EC4Y 0DZ

An Hachette UK Company
www.hachette.co.uk

www.littlebrown.co.uk

For all my clients who have trusted me with
their stories and emotions over the years.

Contents

Part IV: Tools and Strategies for Change

Author's Note

A note before we begin:

The language we use has a powerful influence, and it matters. Research shows that the terms 'overweight' and 'obesity' are stigmatising to those with experience of living in larger bodies. As such, I'll be using words such as 'fat', 'larger bodies' and 'bigger bodies' where possible. When describing the body of a client, I will be using language that we have discussed and they are comfortable with.

All client stories are shared with permission and have been anonymised, modified and merged for confidentiality purposes. The stories are here to bring life to research and bring into sharp focus what so many people think and feel around food and themselves. That is to say, if you see yourself in these stories, it is both deliberate and accidental.

Introduction

Our relationship with food is one of the longest relationships we have in life. We eat several times a day, every day, and we may end up spending more time with food than we do with our families, our partners or our friends. Just like our relationships with people, our connection with food can be easy and enjoyable, or it can feel like a painful and out-of-control rollercoaster that erodes our self-worth.

My job is to help people figure out how they ended up with a relationship with food that feels chaotic or unhealthy, and how they can find peace with food again. Like with any relationship, it can be worked on, and it can get better. That's exactly what we're going to do in this book. The reason you're here with me is to try to understand, and ultimately to improve, your relationship with food.

'Tell me what you eat and I will tell you what you are' said Jean Anthelme Brillat-Savarin, the famous French lawyer and foodie. I want to take this one step further: tell me about what you eat and you'll be telling me about *who* you are, your relationship with yourself, your relationship with others, your culture, your upbringing, your shame and your values. You're telling me about power, control, emotions, identity, love, values, meaning and beliefs. You're telling me a story: the story of you. And so it happens that the more time I spend with people and their relationship with food, the less time we spend talking about food.

All of us make assumptions about others based on what they eat. Research back in the 1980s showed how strong the link is between the foods we eat and how others perceive and judge us for them. People who eat fast food were seen as more religious, health foodies were perceived as more left wing, vegetarians were seen as pacifists, and gourmet diners were seen as liberal and sophisticated people.[1] Sure, this research is a few decades old, but diet-based stereotypes are definitely still alive and well. To bring this into the present day, I've noticed that we are much more likely to think someone who does yoga is also vegan rather than someone who eats a lot of meat, and that someone who lifts weights regularly eats a high-protein diet rather than a plant-based one. I remember seeing media headlines a few years back stating that if you enjoy bitter foods such as gin or dark chocolate, it means that you're more likely to be a sociopath. That is obviously not true at all – the headlines were a total exaggeration of the actual research findings – but if I were to suggest that people who like spicy food are adrenaline junkies and risk takers, you'd probably be inclined to believe me. That's because the basic principle still stands: we make assumptions aplenty about people purely based on their food choices.

Although certain food stereotypes are based on a grain of truth, more often than not the assumptions and judgements we make about what others eat tell us very little about some- one else, and everything about us. When you look over with disgust at a fat person eating a burger, I wonder about your fear of weight gain and what you were taught about how you should look. I wonder what you learned in childhood about your own worth, and whether your parents went on diets. If you hear someone say that they ate two tubs of ice cream in one go and you think: *Just don't have it in the house*, I wonder about your own coping mechanisms for processing difficult emotions, where you learned them from, and if you've ever experienced what it's like to not have enough food.

Most of us have grown up being told two fundamental lies:

1 *There are good foods and bad foods. If I eat the good foods, I'm a good person, if I eat the bad foods, I'm a bad person.*
This may sound drastic, but think about how many times you have heard someone say, 'No thanks, no cake for me, I'm being good today'? or 'I've been so bad today, I've eaten so much chocolate.' We've absorbed this lie of good foods and bad foods so much that we don't even notice how drastic a statement we're making when we say we are a bad person for eating something sweet. We even go so far as to assume these foods have the power to create good bodies and bad bodies, when in reality those don't exist either. These narratives have been instilled in us partly by our pervasive diet culture: a culture that teaches us that our appearance and body shape are more important than our physical and psychological well-being. Diet culture teaches us to value thinness above all else, to reach thinness at all costs, and to equate thinness with goodness.

I want to be very clear: food doesn't have the power to make you a good or bad person, and there are no good or bad foods. All food is context-dependent, always. To one person orange juice is too much sugar, to another it's the only reliable way to ensure that their kids get a portion of fruit and enough vitamin C. Food is always relative; for example, you can die from too little water, or from drinking too much, so is water good or bad? It depends, because context matters.

When I tell people this I often get a defensive reaction and a disbelieving questioning around specific foods. Surely chocolate is bad, or surely sugary drinks – or any other food someone can think of? Just so that you know, I have an answer for every single food someone throws at me, but I don't think a back-and-forth is useful. Instead, I wonder why people are so attached to believing that foods are good or bad, even though this usually isn't helpful at all. Instead of helping, being attached to this narrative usually just produces feelings of guilt and shame.

2 *There are good emotions and bad emotions. If I feel a bad emotion, I must get rid of it or hide it so that no one can see.*
Your typical bad emotion would be something like shame, sadness, anger and jealousy. Like with food, these are emotions that we may be taught are 'bad' and should be avoided. Phrases we hear growing up, like 'Boys don't cry', or 'Don't get angry – you know I hate it', or 'Stop crying or I'll give you something to cry about' teach us to push down these emotions, to avoid them, and we've found plenty of ways to do that very effectively – like using food.

During our lives, we may learn that our emotions are unacceptable, so we use food to cope, either by eating, sometimes to the point of pain and discomfort, or avoiding eating as much as possible. We might use food as a vehicle to change how our bodies – and therefore we as a whole person – are perceived by others. Food is not the problem. Food is an attempted solution to an underlying problem, so we need to figure out the cause of this relationship breakdown, not just treat the symptoms.

Your brain uses food as a coping mechanism because it is trying to help you, not harm you. Food, or any coping mechanisms, may have long-term negative consequences, but in the moment, they are created for a reason, and that reason is because they are *needed*. This, for me, is key to exploring the idea that strategies like emotional eating can be helpful, and to help you understand some possible explanations for the 'why' behind any disordered eating.

There are no bad emotions. All emotions have their place

and can teach us something important. The Pixar movie *Inside Out* is a fantastic example of this, and I often recommend that clients watch it, as it can help to provide language for conversations around emotions, memory, identity and so much more.

The film's principal characters are our basic emotions: joy, sadness, anger, disgust and fear. We observe these characters as they sit behind the control centre in the brain of Riley, who moves house and generally navigates the ups and downs of childhood. While at the beginning Joy tries to stay in charge and dismisses the others, especially Sadness, by the end of the movie it's clear that each of them plays an important role in the story, and in our lives. By the end we see that Joy's desperate bid for positivity and dismissal of Sadness causes great harm, and Sadness becomes crucial for everyone's survival.

Sadness can be painful, but without it we can never experience true joy. Tears feel like a release and can be a signal to others that we need support. There is a moment in *Inside Out* where Joy and Sadness are lost and need the help of their guide. The guide loses something valuable and feels sad, so Joy tries to get him to keep moving and cheer him up by tickling him, pulling faces and suggesting a game. It doesn't work. Then Sadness steps in and says, 'I'm sorry ... they took something that you loved.' Joy sighs and says, 'Sadness, don't make him feel worse', but the guide responds positively to Sadness, feels her support, feels listened to and is able to cry. He then takes a deep breath, declares he feels better and is able to go on with the journey. It's my favourite moment in the whole movie, because it beautifully highlights the incredible value of a so-called 'negative' emotion.

This point extends beyond sadness. Anger tells us about what we perceive as unfair, and it teaches us what we care about. If our boundaries are crossed, if someone hurts a loved one, if we perceive there to be injustice, anger comes up. Anger has a constant undercurrent of hurt, which is why it's often paired with sadness or pain, and why those who have difficulty expressing anger often end up in tears instead.

Fear and disgust both help to keep us safe, they both encourage us away from what can harm and kill us. Fear activates our immediate fight-or-flight response, which enables us to run away from danger. Disgust prevents us from drinking milk that's gone sour, because we smell it and immediately feel repulsed by it, thereby protecting us from potential food poisoning. All these emotions have a function, and we can't choose to feel some emotions and not others.

Our emotions are important teachers. The stronger the emotion, the more likely it is that the event, experience, or person provoking it, holds *meaning* for us. This can be through a positive and encouraging experience or a difficult and traumatic one. Meaning is individual and personal.

Our food experiences hold incredible meaning for us. We believe that we are what we eat, as the food we eat becomes our various organs and tissues. Food is one of the most powerful metaphors we have, so it's perhaps not surprising that food and emotions are so linked. I often see people who are so proficient at denying their pain or minimising their experiences in life that they believe their problems about food are *only* problems about food. It is surface level, like the tip of the iceberg denying the existence of everything below the waterline. When people feel that they are suffering with their relationship with food, they believe that solving the problem of food will mean everything else in their life falls into place. I am reminded of the gay man with internalised homophobia who is so afraid of his shame that he keeps bringing the conversation back to what he ate last weekend; of the malnourished and traumatised young woman who asks me every week 'Are you sure it's OK for me to eat this much food?' every time we talk about her father; of the career-driven professional who says she cannot date until she has lost weight, and brushes away her abusive ex as 'ancient history'.

We will not be staying at the surface in this book; we will be exploring the entire iceberg, not just what is visible above the surface. Otherwise, we are doing ourselves a disservice.

When I first started working as a nutritionist, I assumed that I'd be seeing clients who are simply looking to be healthier, who had read pieces of misinformation on social media and wanted reassurance. I assumed I'd be asking for food diaries and performing nutritional analyses of the macro- and micronutrients that they were consuming day to day – that very quickly turned out not to be the case. The people coming my way often showed signs of deeper emotional issues, hints of trauma that would spill out in later sessions, and layers of food rules piled on top of a deep-rooted shame. I could sense these revelations bubbling below the surface, sometimes overflowing through tearful stories about their childhood experiences, and I knew all I was qualified to do was listen. That had to be enough. But it wasn't.

Most people who come to see me in clinic do so because they want a better relationship with food. When I outline my process to them, I describe it as a little bit like a doctor's appointment and a lot like therapy, or simply as 'food therapy'. In truth, what they can expect depends on what they bring to the sessions. Yes, we'll talk about food and what they eat, but we'll spend far more time on the *why*. People come to me because of their issues with food, but we can very easily spend weeks on end barely mentioning food at all. Often, someone's behaviour and beliefs around food are an indicator of who they are as a person, their childhood experiences, their emotional regulation, and what they've been taught about themselves. Food is simply the obvious symptom of a deeper emotional problem, so they search for a nutritionist, and get a food therapist.

There are only a handful of people in the UK who have

qualifications in both nutrition and psychotherapy. I am one of them. I trained in nutrition first, getting a masters degree in London, then followed that with training in intuitive eating, body image and disordered eating. I qualified in acceptance and commitment therapy (ACT) and CBT for eating disorders (CBT-E), before taking the plunge into further training to become an accredited psychotherapist and counsellor. I am one of only a handful of people in the UK who bridges the gap between food and therapy.

I see clients on a one-to-one basis in my clinic in London and virtually around the world. My clients have shaped my work immensely, which is why I share some of their stories here.

The stories we tell ourselves matter. As humans, we respond far more to stories than we do to facts. The people I see often have a difficult relationship with food. Some have never been to therapy before (and express no interest in it), others have had therapy in the past but want to see someone who understands nutrition. I see people who, for one reason or another, can't or won't get an eating disorder diagnosis, and end up slipping through the cracks of the healthcare system.

These people come to me. We spend months, sometimes years, engaging in 'food therapy' as I try to help them understand themselves better and feel more comfortable around food. We talk about food, and so much more. Their experiences have shaped my practice, and, with their permission, I'd like to share some of their stories in this book, because each story is important.

Ultimately, I don't believe in 'fixing' emotional eating by resolving to never eat when we're stressed, or bored, or angry, or sad or lonely. We often eat because we are hungry, not for food, but for something that is missing in our lives. I don't believe that disordered and restrictive eating can be resolved without looking deeper into the reasons why we got here. I want to help you understand your 'why', work out what you're really hungry for, and help you see that this is about more than just food.

How to use this book

This book is divided into four sections. First, we will establish what your relationship with food is like, not because you need a label but to encourage you to explore where you are right now and begin the process of holding up a mirror to your own experience. Then we'll explore the common origins of food issues that I see in clinic. Food is complex, and although for some there might be a single significant event in life, for many it will be a series of intertwined factors that have led them to have a poor relationship with food. After that we'll move on to the barriers that may be preventing you from having or pursuing a better relationship with food and yourself. Finally, we will explore tools and strategies you may wish to implement for yourself. I encourage you not to skip ahead to this section, because often it's only once we know how we got here *and* what's in our way that we can look to solutions. We pause, we notice, we get curious, and then we move forward.

Hold these questions in your mind as we continue:

- How would I describe my relationship with food?
- Where did I learn this relationship with food? (Origins)
- What's stopping me from developing a greater relationship with food? (Barriers)
- What can I do to change this? (Solutions)
- What is my food story?

Are you ready to be curious?

PART I

FOOD AND YOU

1

Setting the Scene

When a new client sits down on the large soft armchair opposite me, I start the session by saying, 'Tell me about why we're meeting here today.' It's an open invitation to tell their story in a way that makes sense to them. It may not be the most concise, connected or chronological story, but it is their story as it appears in their mind, unrehearsed and raw, which is exactly how I want to hear it.

If I had to describe the people I meet and their relationship with food, they broadly fit into one or more categories: disordered eating, emotional eating, chronic dieting, and body image concerns. These are by no means separate boxes; there is considerable overlap here, and for most clients of mine at least two of these apply; for example, someone in her thirties may have been dieting since she was twelve years old, has a whole series of conflicting food rules in her head that she can't shake, eats to cope with stress and anxiety, and feels disgust towards her body.

Although I may notice patterns in people, I'm not interested in giving them a label – I am interested in the story they have to tell. If someone has found a label that they feel applies and holds meaning to them, that's their experience and their choice, and I will always respect that. I have used the categories below in case they resonate with you and help you to find the language to tell your own story. As you read, notice what jumps out at you and connects with you.

Disordered eating

All eating exists on a continuum; on the one end we have 'normal' eating which doesn't take up a lot of headspace, is not anxiety-inducing, is flexible, fits in with a social life, and feels good in that person's body. On the other end we have an eating disorder that is clinically significant to the point where a diagnosis can be applied. Between those two arbitrary lines we have disordered eating. But where does normal eating end and disordered eating begin? It is tricky to pin down. I would say when anxiety around eating comes into the picture, but even there I can think of exceptions: if you have allergies, eating out at a restaurant might make you feel nervous due to the risk this may present, especially if you've had bad experiences in the past. Where does disordered eating become an eating disorder? Well, as with all psychological disorders, some old guys in an office somewhere came up with a series of diagnostic criteria, wrote them down back in 1952, and if you tick the boxes, voila – you get a diagnosis! Today, you can access treatment (or at least join the months-long waiting list). Often whether you get a diagnosis or not is dictated by your body mass index (BMI), even though eating disorders are psychological disorders at their core. We pay more attention to the physical consequences of eating disorders than we do to their actual psychological presentation, to the point where we have a separate diagnosis for anorexia nervosa and 'atypical' anorexia – the latter being anorexia with a hefty serving of fatphobia. Many people are unable to get a diagnosis for exactly this reason: their BMI is deemed too high. It's an unfortunate effect of the system. In my view, the priorities are the wrong way round. While physical health does, at times, need to take priority due to a very real risk of danger or death, this only resolves the most obvious symptom of an eating disorder, not the underlying issues. True recovery is only achieved when there is enough relief from the psychological components of an eating disorder to live a normal life and feel calm around food. In a nutshell, then, while an eating disorder is a diagnosis, disordered eating is a descriptive phrase. For me, in my practice, I don't need a diagnosis to work with someone. I don't give out diagnoses either; I work with the story someone tells me. For this reason, I'm using 'disordered eating' here as an umbrella term that includes eating disorders, but also recognises those unable or unwilling to get a diagnosis. I see all your experiences as valid.

Signs and symptoms that you might have disordered eating are: anxiety around specific foods, chronic weight fluctuations, rigid rituals around foods or food situations, feelings of guilt or shame after eating, engaging in compensatory behaviours after eating forbidden foods, and a preoccupation with weight and shape.

Some side effects of disordered eating include anxiety, depression, low self-esteem, food obsession, not being able to change the world because you're too busy thinking about how you look and what you're eating, malnutrition, nutrient deficiencies and osteoporosis.

Potential signs of disordered eating

- Anxiety around specific foods or food situations (such as spontaneous dinner plans).

➡

- Spending a lot of time checking food labels.
- Rigid rituals and routines surrounding food and exercise.
- Feelings of guilt and shame associated with eating.
- Preoccupation with food, weight and body image that negatively impacts quality of life.
- A feeling of loss of control around food.
- Using exercise, food restriction, fasting or purging to 'make up for' eating certain foods.
- Food dictating how good/bad you feel about yourself that day.

Emotional eating

Emotional eating is a heavily misunderstood subject. A quick Google search on emotional eating brings up article after article on 'How to stop emotional eating', as if that's something that's even feasible or desirable. This is the wrong approach. Hear me out: to be an emotional eater is to be human. It's a tool so many of us use because it works. When we get dumped, we go full Bridget Jones with a tub of ice cream; when we're stressed, we eat chocolate; when we feel sad, we order pizza; when we feel homesick, we eat foods that remind us of home. These are normal responses to normal emotions. But, of course, as with all things, there comes a point where every helpful thing becomes harmful, where we become so reliant on food as a way of coping that it encourages emotional dysregulation, and where it causes problems.

Emotional eating is a subject that is generally explored and discussed in the context of overeating and weight gain. I find this incredibly boring. It reduces a nuanced human behaviour to a matter of aesthetics, into something that contributes to a non-contagious 'epidemic' of bodies society deems not good enough. We assume that emotional eating = overeating = weight gain = bad. Even research on the subject often begins with a sentence on how emotional eating (which is defined as eating in response to negative emotions), is a dysregulated physiological response to feeling intense emotions, because it differs from the 'typical' human response – namely to lose your appetite when you feel sad. I have questions already: what about positive emotions? We don't just eat in response to negative ones. Why are we assuming the emotion is intense? Why are we assuming that all bodies react the same way to emotions? Not everyone loses their appetite. Why are we even assuming that emotional eating must mean overeating? That certainly hasn't been my experience. Most importantly: why are we simply labelling this as bad without attempting to understand *why* it happens in the first place?

There are actually several types of emotional eating that exist on a spectrum. On the most benign end we have eating for pleasure. Not hunger, just pleasure. I would argue that many of us do this on a regular basis. Food is supposed to taste good, and it is pleasurable to bask in its glory. Next up we have eating for comfort. Isn't it wonderful that food can offer us comfort in times where little else is available? That warm feeling of a full stomach is often associated with comfort and safety and contentment. It's an effective short-term antidote to emptiness. Heading in the destructive direction next is eating for distraction. This can be alleviation from boredom, to distract from uncomfortable thoughts or feelings, or simply for something to do. Next to that we have eating for sedation, to avoid feeling. When emotions are tough or deemed unacceptable, food helps to push those down so that we don't have to feel any of them – effective in the short-term, not in the long-term, that is. Finally, the most destructive form of emotional eating is eating for punishment. It is eating because you believe you have done something wrong and deserve to suffer the consequences. It is a form of self-harm, often driven by self-hatred.

Research on emotional eating is relatively recent and is largely confusing and unhelpful. There are a number of emotional eating quizzes and scoring systems available and yet none of them seem to actually reliably measure emotional eating.[2] Focusing on the more destructive end of the emotional eating spectrum, the end I'm most likely to see in clinic, my simplified definition of emotional eating is this: eating in response to emotions that are deemed to be 'wrong' in some way, and therefore need to be avoided. Eating pushes those emotions down so that they don't have to be felt.

Ultimately, when someone tells me that they are an emotional eater I try not to make assumptions. Instead, I want to understand what this particular person sitting in front of me right now in this moment means by emotional eating. I want them to give me their definition and their understanding of what is going on in their life and in their body. I use their understanding as a starting point and go from there. At least then we can begin on the same page.

When it comes to emotional eating, the problem is not the food. The problem is that emotions are being avoided. Food is the solution. It's no different from using alcohol, drugs, cleaning, work or exercise as a distraction or suppression tool. These coping mechanisms are not inherently 'bad'. They are either helpful or unhelpful, and their helpfulness can change with time. In a nutshell, emotional eating can be an attempt to solve a symbolic, metaphorical hunger with physical fullness.

Potential signs of emotional eating

- Eating when feeling stressed/sad/angry/bored/lonely/anxious.
- Eating in order to redirect/change an emotion.
- Eating to numb an emotion.
- Seeking solace and comfort in food.
- Eating without really understanding why you're eating.
- Feeling guilt and shame after turning to food.
- Eating when not physically hungry.

Chronic dieting

Our diet culture society teaches us that if our bodies take up too much space we must shrink them, for our health, our happiness, success and to be seen as attractive by others. We are told we have to go on a diet, any diet, as long as it works and makes us smaller. For some people, this seems to work. For the vast majority, each diet cycle, each period of losing weight and gaining it back, leaves them heavier than before.

I see many chronic dieters in clinic, some who have been dieting since they were eight or nine years old and are now sick of restriction. Sometimes we have to do something ten times over before we pause and consider that there might be another way; a way of living that doesn't involve a restrictive diet with food rules. I don't work with weight loss; I don't offer any restrictive plans or offer any advice to shed the pounds. People know this when they come to see me; in fact, it's exactly the reason why they come to see me. Dieting hasn't worked for them, and they're ready for something new, even if the idea of giving up dieting is a terrifying prospect.

Whether chronic dieting is a form of disordered eating or not is up for debate. I wouldn't go so far as to say that every single diet is a form of disordered eating, but the chronic, repeating nature of it feels different to me. To some, there is a sense of madness to it – trying the same thing over and over again expecting a different result – all the while being on the receiving end of pressures from society to keep trying in order to look a certain way. Plus, there's the anxiety that can come with going on diet after diet and not knowing whether the restaurant your friends have chosen has dishes that you're allowed to eat, or having the fun taken out of the evening because you're calculating points or calories.

If you find yourself going on a diet, losing some weight, regaining it again, only to start the cycle all over again soon after, you're experiencing what's known as weight cycling. While this has the perceived benefit of 'at least people won't think I'm lazy and not trying', it carries its own health risks, particularly to mental health, as those who weight cycle tend to have poorer mental health than those who stay the same weight, including at a higher weight. There is also emerging evidence to suggest that weight cycling increases your risk of heart disease.[3]

In my experience, I often hear people saying that they don't want to *want to* diet. They feel that they *should* diet because that's what's expected of them, but they're tired of it. They want to try something different, but they're afraid, creating this push and pull between desire and fear. Sometimes the familiar and miserable feels safer than the unknown. In the end, you just have to take the leap. The fact that you're reading this suggests that you're probably ready. Maybe it's time.

Potential signs that you're ready to stop dieting

- You're fed up with dieting.
- You can recognise that dieting hasn't worked for you long term.
- You find yourself unable to 'stick to' a diet for as long as you used to.
- You don't have much hope that another diet will work.
- You don't want to diet but aren't sure what else you could do.
- You don't want to diet but you're afraid of what might happen if you don't diet.
- You don't want your children to see you dieting.

Body image concerns

Body image is defined as the thoughts, feelings, perceptions and beliefs that make up the way we feel about our bodies. It is our subjective experience of being 'in' our body. Poor body image, or body dissatisfaction, is depressingly common, appearing in younger and younger children, and it can last someone's entire life. It is characterised by pessimism, negative self-talk, lack of acceptance, comparison and shame. It can manifest in the form of mirror-checking, poking and prodding body parts, not being able to accept compliments, and disordered eating.

We live in a society that equates health with the way we look, and our appearance with our worth. We attach a huge number of assumptions and judgements of morality and worth to a body, which places us under enormous pressure to exist within a very narrow framework of beauty, desirability and health. This standard of beauty is unachievable for the majority of the population.

Body image concerns and food concerns tend to go hand in hand. After all, the food we eat becomes our various organs and tissues and cells. Negative body image is a key part of (and a predictor of) a variety of health issues such as depression, eating disorders and body dysmorphic disorder.* People who are dissatisfied with their bodies are more likely to engage in unhealthy and unhelpful eating behaviours, and are less likely to take care of themselves.

Positive body image, on the other hand, is not merely the absence of negative body image. It is also not as simple as feeling great about your body 24/7, every day of the year. That's a little unrealistic. Positive body image includes optimism, self-esteem, adaptive coping and resilience, acceptance of the body regardless of weight or perceived imperfections, and respect of the body by engaging in health-promoting behaviours. When I have witnessed people put this into practice, they are so much more content with themselves.

At this point you may be thinking: *Well, if I lose weight, I'll have better body image.* I'm afraid that it's a bit more complex than that. Firstly, yes, the world will treat you better if you're in a smaller body. You're less likely to be harassed on the street, more likely to be hired, more likely to find a partner, and more likely to have healthcare professionals actually listen to your concerns rather than blame everything on your weight.[4] The world is easier to navigate if you're not fat, and you can't just love yourself out of discrimination. Having said that, body image is complex, and the way that others perceive us and treat us is just one component of it. I have seen too many people despair when they tell me that when their body was bigger they didn't

---

* Body dysmorphic disorder is an anxiety disorder related to body image, where a person becomes fixated on perceived flaws about their appearance, to the extent that it disrupts someone's daily life.

like it, when their body was smaller they still didn't like it, and now that it's bigger again they definitely don't like it. Their body changes, but the negative view they have of their bodies doesn't. To me, that sends a message loud and clear: *it's not about how your body looks.* The change doesn't need to be aesthetic – it needs to be internal, in your mind, through understanding, acceptance and compassion.

One of the reasons I want to introduce body image here is because emotions can be stored in the body and can produce a physical reaction; for example, asthma is fifty times more prevalent in traumatised children than their non-traumatised peers.[5] IBS (irritable bowel syndrome) symptoms are common in people with eating disorders, particularly during recovery, partly because of the stress and anxiety around eating. Anxiety can feel like gut pain, or it can feel like someone is squeezing your lungs. Shock can feel like a punch in the stomach. Stress can feel like a weight on your shoulders, and grief like someone is crushing your heart. Some of this originates in the fight-or-flight response, where acute stress causes an increased heart rate, dilated pupils and muscle activation. Some of it also links to the gut–brain axis: our two-way communication between the gut and the brain that helps explain why we get 'butter-flies' in our stomach when we feel nervous. But it goes beyond this: researchers have mapped which locations in the body are activated when we feel certain emotions, and the patterns are surprisingly consistent between individuals.[6] Although we don't fully understand why, our bodies can help us to identify and understand what we're feeling.

When we use food to soothe or push away our emotions, we literally and symbolically push our feelings down with food into our stomachs to be digested. That feeling of blood rushing to the stomach and gut to focus on digestion can feel warm and comforting, but it can also feel painful when we've eaten too much. Because we feel this pain in our body, we see our bloated stomachs in the mirror, we remember our hands manoeuvring the food into our mouths, we then blame our bodies. Our body becomes the scapegoat, the stage on which our shameful act of eating is played out and witnessed by others. Our body becomes the thing that is judged.

Signs of negative body image

- You don't respect your body.
- You feel bad about your body.
- You feel that your body has few or no good qualities.
- You feel embarrassed about/ashamed of your body.
- You try to ignore your body's needs.
- Your behaviour reveals your negative attitude towards your body; for example, you cover up even in summer, your posture is hunched over, you try to avoid looking at your body.
- You are uncomfortable in your body.
- You regularly compare your body to others.

Now you have a sense of where your relationship with food is right now, as well as your body image. You have the language to describe it (should you choose to use the terms above) and hopefully a sense that your situation is not unique, but depressingly common. You have your answer to our first important question: 'How would I describe my relationship with food?'

It's time to now take this forward as we move on to our next question: 'Where did I learn this relationship with food?' It's time to delve into where all this has come from so that we can add to your understanding of your food story.

PART II

THE ORIGINS OF FOOD ISSUES

2

Trauma

When writer Roxane Gay experienced a significant traumatic event in her childhood, her response was to eat. In her powerful memoir *Hunger,* she writes that she ate 'to build my body into a fortress'.

I understand her perfectly.

Trauma types: 'big T' and 'little t'

Trauma is a psychological and emotional response to a severely distressing or disturbing experience. Sometimes, the experience can shape our lives forever and leave long-term marks on our psyche. Although we may have broad 'official' ideas of what is and isn't trauma, in my experience it is heavily individual. If you experience something as traumatic, it is real, and I believe you completely. In psychology we also sometimes refer to 'big T' and 'little t' trauma. The 'big T' covers experiences that are often associated with PTSD (post-traumatic stress disorder) such as sexual violence, physical abuse and life-threatening situations like natural disasters. 'Little t' traumas don't typically meet the criteria for PTSD but are still valid and can be life altering. This can include bullying, emotional abuse and difficult breakups. For some people, repeated exposure to 'little t' traumas can cause more harm than a single 'big T' trauma.

In my clinic, I generally see two types of people who have experienced trauma in life. The first comes in with a clear story: I experienced trauma and now my relationship with food is like this. The second sit down and tell a story of food, then five minutes before the end they shuffle awkwardly, look at the clock, and say, 'I'm not sure if it's even relevant, but …' and that piece of the puzzle emerges. On the surface, they see no real connection between these events, and yet there is a gut feeling that this is important information to share. Every one of these people comes to me to discuss food, and every time we have ended up discussing so much more.

When Roger was a child, his father would beat him severely for any perceived 'mistake' or anything he deemed 'not good enough'. If he expressed anger, stood up for his mother, if his grades weren't perfect or he made a sound his father didn't like, he was punished. Alongside this, he was constantly told that everything he did wasn't good enough, selfless enough, quiet enough. This is clearly physical and emotional abuse, but to him it was simply his 'normal'. Roger internalised the idea that he was a terrible person who didn't deserve anything good, who couldn't trust anyone, who didn't deserve food. He had been taught from a young age that depriving himself of food was an appropriate and necessary form of self-punishment and that his emotions had to be suppressed, as expressing them was unsafe. There was a total disconnect between his brain and his body. His response to this enduring trauma, eighteen years of it, was to eat as little as possible to make himself as small as possible, to make himself less of a target.

There is no one typical response to trauma. Often, the responses we do have are not conscious, they happen seemingly out of our control. Roger didn't decide to starve himself: his behaviour was a continuation of the beliefs he had internalised as a child that said, 'you don't deserve this'. It was his brain's way of keeping him safe.

The way we respond to trauma is incredibly complex. I stand firmly in the belief that the brain is not self-destructive, your brain is always trying to help you. Brains are problem-solving machines, and in response to the problem of a traumatic event, the brain might do all sorts of things that seem strange to us in order to try to provide a solution. For Roger, not eating was an effective solution that had (ironically) kept him alive. He had shut off from his entire body, not feeling cold or pain, or emotions beyond extremes. He would walk in snow with no gloves, not notice his hand burning if he spilled hot coffee on it, and suppress years of painful memories. He kept his body in a state of simply surviving, where it had neither the means nor motive to process what had happened to him. He could avoid all the pain and hurt he had experienced . . . in the short term.

To an outsider, it looks as if Roger was self-destructing. To me, it looks like he was doing the best he could with an incredibly limited toolbox and an internal narrative that said he was worthless.

Think of it this way: remember the last time you accidently sat on your foot for too long and it fell asleep? It goes numb, totally numb, as though it's disconnected from the rest of you. You feel nothing. Then you release the pressure, blood starts flowing back through and you experience pins and needles. This is not a fun experience; it can even be quite painful. At this point you have one of two options: sit back on your foot so that it goes numb again, or go through the pain and discomfort of pins and needles until your foot feels normal again. It can be so tempting to sit on it again, to go back to the lack of feeling, but if you do, you know it can't last forever. Eventually you're going to have to go straight through the centre of the pain.

This response to trauma allows us to suppress our emotions and memories, our pain, our suffering. It allows us to get on with life rather than being consumed by our experiences. *It is your brain trying to be helpful.* Even if in the moment it doesn't feel helpful.

Chloe experienced sexual assault as a teenager. Even years later, she would wake up almost every night in a panic from nightmares. She found purging helped to remove the memory from her body – a solution that is both visceral and highly symbolic. She worked hard in therapy to stop the purging behaviour, which then morphed into a different solution. Now, the only thing that consistently helps her bring her nervous system down and go back to sleep is chocolate milk. She has a cup, more if she needs it, and feels a sense of calm as soon as she notices it sliding down her throat. It's instantaneous and highly effective – it works every single time. Why is this such a powerful solution for her? She says she feels 'heavier', as if she's put on a weighted blanket. She says, 'Chocolate milk is someone holding me and saying it's going to be OK.' Although this worked in the moment, the next morning she would wake up feeling disgust at herself, which would linger throughout the day. Following one of our early discussions, she tried gargling mouthwash after drinking chocolate milk, which I suggested to see what would happen if she woke up without the traces of chocolate milk in her mouth. My hope was that it might break the cycle of disgust, and it did. It also meant so much more to her than that, as it held huge symbolic significance in the form of cleanliness, control and getting rid of any traces of something (or someone) that wasn't her.

To me it is totally understandable that someone who has been raped or sexually assaulted would go to great lengths to 'purge' the other person from themselves, including the memory of that person. This could be like Chloe, in the form of vomiting and feeling empty, or in the form of 'purging' the version of yourself you used to be, and building your body into a fortress. Shale had experienced multiple sexual assaults in their teenage years, always after they had been on a diet and lost weight. They made a connection between being in a smaller body and unwanted attention from men, on a totally unconscious level, and avoided dieting ever since. It wasn't until they opened up and talked this through in therapy that this association became conscious in a sudden moment of awareness. When we factored in their internalised fatphobia, and their belief that thin bodies are more desirable than fat bodies (thanks to diet culture), they were able to make sense of their experiences.

The food connection

As someone who is both a therapist and a nutrition professional, I can clearly see why so many traumatic experiences manifest themselves through food. Food is an incredibly powerful metaphor that carries so much meaning in life. When we feel as if we're not enough, food can fill us up. When we feel as if we're too much, purging can bring us back down. These behaviours help us to regulate our sense of self in a way that we feel we can control. Looking to the research, one analysis of 57,000 women found that those who experienced physical or sexual abuse as children were twice as likely to have issues they described as overeating.[7]

These examples are what we would describe as 'big T' trauma: hugely significant life events that have changed someone at the core of who they understand themselves to be. Sometimes, however, trauma can be more subtle.

Marina has one clear memory from her childhood that stands out to her above all others. After her parents filed for divorce, she remembers her father saying to her, 'I had to divorce your mother, she's gained so much weight.' Shortly after, Marina dropped out of sports teams at school. At the time these two events seemed totally unrelated to her, but with the power of hindsight and curiosity she's able to connect the dots: she wanted to defend her mother and spite her father. She had started therapy because her boyfriend had threatened to break up with her if she continued to gain weight, and it had brought back all the painful memories from her childhood. As a therapist I'm not supposed to judge, but in my head I was thinking: *What an asshole.* A few sessions in she triumphantly announced that she'd ditched him.

The parallel in experience here was so great that her current relationship situation brought back all the emotions and memories associated with a past event, so much so that for Marina it felt as if it were happening in the present moment. This is sometimes described as a trauma response: a trigger that leads the brain to merge the past and present. The distress Marina experienced from this merging of past and present led her to eat *more* to soothe herself, and produced a great deal of anxiety.

Sometimes the reason someone enters therapy, the presenting problem, ends up being very different from the real problem that person wants to solve. When Winona first signed up for online sessions, she described feeling anxiety, a worry that she overeats, and uncertainty about her relationship. She had linked her food concerns with an experience in early adulthood where she had dated someone who struggled with bulimia. She was able to trace the origins of her food anxiety back to this experience. Now, I'm not a die-hard Freudian who believes that everything always stems from childhood, but I do find it a useful topic to bring up to understand someone's early environment better. I asked her about her food experiences growing up, and she said, 'We always had enough food, even though my parents were both drug addicts and forgot to cook, they always ensured there were enough ready meals in the house.' In her case, because she hadn't experienced any food insecurity or deprivation, she hadn't made any connection between these experiences and her relationship with food now. She asked, 'Do you think it's connected?' (a question I'm asked a lot). My answer is always, 'I'm not sure. I can see how it might be, but I don't know enough about you to give you a clear yes or no. We can discuss it, though, to understand your experiences better, and if you decide that it's connected, then it's connected.'

While Winona hadn't experienced any obvious neglect, there was a subtler element to her experience, which was having to parent herself from a young age. That is a huge amount of responsibility to give a young child, and it can lead them to grow up quicker than their peers. Her parents were loving and cared about her deeply, but their addiction prevented them from being the parents Winona needed them to be.

Similarly, Hazel grew up with an alcoholic father, and learned early on to mould herself according to his state and needs. She internalised the idea that if she could just be the 'right' version of herself for him, he wouldn't shout at her or dismiss her, but instead engage with her. This is quite a common experience with parents who are unable to provide the consistency that children benefit from. The child ends up trying to control the situation in any way they can, because they reach towards the idea that they are the cause of it, because the complexity of alcoholism, or any addiction or psychological illness, is far more difficult for the young brain to understand. They become the ultimate people-pleasers, which in Hazel's case meant she grew up with no solid sense of self, few ambitions and few desires for herself.

Research examining the link between trauma and disordered eating has come up with three possible links. Firstly, trauma often leaves people feeling highly negative about themselves, with beliefs of being 'broken' or 'not good enough'. When people hold these negative core beliefs about themselves, they are more likely to engage in destructive behaviours or simply not pursue health-promoting behaviours. Secondly, emotional eating (either eating or avoiding eating in response to emotions) can provide short-term relief from trauma-related negative thoughts and feelings. Thirdly, disordered eating can provide a means to avoid unwanted attention from past and potential future perpetrators of trauma – this is especially the case when someone has experienced sexual trauma.[8]

Identifying the core

How someone responds to trauma, whether someone tends towards overeating or undereating as a result of traumatic experiences, is impossible to predict. It is only with the power of hindsight that we can connect the dots and clearly see the picture of their relationship with food. The common theme, however, is that trauma leaves people with feelings of shame, feelings of worthlessness, feelings of being broken, feelings of being not good enough and not deserving of good things in life. These beliefs have far-reaching impacts throughout someone's life. They constantly sit beneath the surface, underpinning so much of how we behave. But the situation is far from hopeless. No one is born feeling they are not good enough. We are born with an inherent sense of our own worth. We are born the centre of our own universes. It is through our experiences in life, particularly our relationships with others, and what we learn from those experiences and relationships, that we begin to believe that we are not good enough. If we can learn it, that means we can also unlearn it, and there is great power and hope in that.

In my experience, it can be hard to identify feeling not good enough. It is incredibly uncomfortable to say out loud, 'I'm not good enough', and we can struggle to connect this to our food behaviours. The way I describe this to my clients and encourage them to picture this is a ladder that we climb down rung by rung.

On the surface, like the earth's crust, there is the behaviour – there is food. This is the top rung. At the centre, in the molten core, there is the core belief, the bottom of the ladder. When we put them next to each other, they don't seem connected at all. But as we climb down the 'if–then' ladder of self-awareness, gradually unveiling deeper after deeper layer of someone's sense of self, the connections become apparent.

Let me offer you an example: we might start with, 'I eat too much'. From there, we climb down each rung by asking, 'If this is true, then what does this mean?' until we reach the core belief at the centre.

- I eat too much.
- If I eat too much, then it means I'm greedy.
- If I am greedy, then I'm taking more than I deserve.
- If I'm taking more than I deserve, then I'm a bad person.
- If I'm a bad person, then I'm not good enough.

When we connect the top and bottom rung, we get: 'If I eat too much, then I'm not good enough'.

We can step down this ladder with almost any belief system. Let's take a belief about the body as another example.

- My body was better when it was smaller.
- If my body was better smaller, then my body now is not attractive enough.
- If my body isn't attractive enough, I won't find a partner.
- If I can't find a partner, I will be alone forever.
- If I'm alone forever, then I am unlovable.

When we connect the top and bottom rung here, we see that the way someone views their body is clearly connected to their core belief of being unlovable.

The 'if–then' ladder can be both incredibly revealing and also painful for people. When I go through this process with people in clinic, often there is hopelessness, or people can get stuck in a loop that prevents them from reaching the core because it's just too uncomfortable. I recommend giving this a try for yourself, tracking down the steps of the ladder, to see where you end up. If you feel discomfort, you're probably getting close. If you find yourself getting stuck, that's OK. Take a break, and come back to it another day, or return to it with the help of a therapist to guide you and provide support. Identifying your core belief about yourself isn't compulsory, but I have seen it provide such illumination for people, like a light-bulb moment, that it has become a tool I use incredibly often.

Going through this process often brings up so many questions, questions you might be asking right now. How can I possibly change a core belief about myself? How can I do a 180 from 'I'm not good enough' to 'I am good enough'? It sounds like an overwhelming challenge. And I totally understand that. The beautiful thing about this ladder is that every rung is an opportunity for change. Every rung has the opportunity to be challenged and broken. I find that incredibly hopeful.

It is so tempting to minimise the difficult experiences we've had in life, to say 'every family has problems'. Of course they do, but there is an ocean of difference between family problems and experiencing trauma. British paediatrician and psychoanalyst Donald Winnicott coined the term 'good enough mother' to recognise that while children have important needs that need to be met, a parent doesn't have to be perfect or get everything right to raise psychologically healthy children. A 'good enough' parent responds quickly, empathically and consistently, and encourages the expression of a range of emotions. With 'good enough' caregivers, children learn that they are safe, that wounds can be healed and mistakes can be learned from. When their parents screw up (because everyone does), they make amends – they apologise. If a child learns that they are not safe, that everything is their fault, that their needs won't be met, then that child learns to expect pain and rejection from others. Bessel van der Kolk, author of the incredibly popular book *The Body Keeps the Score*, says, 'We get our first lessons in self care from how we are cared for by others. Children whose parents are reliable sources of comfort and strength have a lifetime advantage. A kind of buffer against the worst that fate can hand them.'

The brain of a child cannot cope with the notion that their parents, the very people who are supposed to be their protectors and caregivers, are incapable of looking after them and meeting their needs. It's a thought that is simply too devastating for the brain of a child to handle, so the brain rejects it. Rather than accepting that their parents are unable to care for them in the way they need for healthy development, the child blames themselves and assumes that there must be something they did wrong or something they did to deserve this. The blame is internalised every time because that is the only way the brain can continue on. This is then the foundation on which that child's self-worth is built. It is awful and painful, and deeply unfair.

Traumatic experiences have far-reaching impacts on our lives, affecting our beliefs, thoughts and behaviours. This can show up with food, through using food to soothe or punish or suppress emotions and memories. It can also show up in an inability to maintain romantic relationships, a lack of trust, difficulty regulating emotions, difficulty sleeping, substance misuse, avoidance, depression, anxiety, dissociation, and more. Situations that seem benign to others may trigger a fight-or-flight response, where your body and nervous system are on high alert and you feel unsafe.

The window of tolerance

Traumatic stress tends to evoke two emotional extremes: feeling either too much emotion (overwhelm) or too little (numb). The space between these two states is known as our 'window of tolerance' – a term coined by Dr Dan Siegel. Within this window lies the range of emotional intensity and variety of experiences that our nervous system can handle safely. Our nervous system is built to handle fluctuations between activation (the sympathetic nervous system) and settling (the parasympathetic nervous system). Each fluctuation brings us closer to the upper or lower limits of our window of tolerance but, day to day, someone who hasn't experienced trauma will be able to navigate this and have clear coping mechanisms when they get close to the edge.

If you have experienced trauma, your window of tolerance might be narrower compared to someone who hasn't experienced trauma. This means that you will often experience activation beyond the typical gentle ebb and flow due to triggers, or you will find that even the slightest activation above normal hits the edge of your window of tolerance and causes overwhelm. This is important, because someone standing right next to you might react with a disinterested shrug to something that your nervous system struggles to cope with. Everyone's window of tolerance is slightly different: the exact same level of arousal and activation can bring one person to a comfortable place within their window of tolerance but take a second person over the edge. I often hear people with trauma say that they feel 'crazy' around their non-traumatised friends, simply because they react so differently. You're not crazy; you have a narrow window of tolerance.

Beyond the upper limit of our window of tolerance (hyperarousal) we experience anxiety, fear, emotional flooding and panic. This state impacts our ability to eat and sleep normally, and may make going about our normal daily life incredibly challenging. In some people it leads to a paralysing inability to do anything. Hyperarousal is the body's way of staying prepared and ready for threats, which can persist years after trauma occurs. It is also one of the main diagnostic criteria for PTSD.

Even though hyperarousal is a method of self-protection it can also have harmful effects in that it can interfere with someone's ability to take their time to assess and respond in an appropriate manner to stimuli around them, like sudden movements or loud noises. Roger's traumatic experiences with his father meant that even the sound of footsteps in the flat above him could trigger him into a state of hyperarousal and panic that to an outsider would seem nonsensical. Essentially, the nervous system is reacting as if there is danger even though there is none. It can take time to work through the worldview that life is unsafe and danger is hiding everywhere.

Hypoarousal is the opposite; it's a state of shutting down, disconnecting, dissociating and numbness. This can happen immediately following hyperarousal as the brain shuts off in order to cope, as our bodies struggle to stay in one state for too long. Some individuals with trauma will find themselves spending a lot of time fluctuating between hyperarousal and hypoarousal, with very little time spent within the window of tolerance. If you think this sounds exhausting, you're absolutely right.

In my experience, when I describe the concept of the window of tolerance to my clients it can be incredibly grounding, and it can help people to realise that they're not 'broken' or 'overreacting', their nervous system is having an understandable response given past experiences and events. But that doesn't mean things have to stay that way. It is possible to widen your own window of tolerance.

Hyperarousal is often associated with fight or flight, but there are actually four stress or trauma responses: fight, flight, freeze and fawn. Fight usually involves aggression and conflict; flight involves getting away as quickly as possible. Freezing means becoming incapable of engaging or making a decision. And the fawn response is about pleasing, over-apologising and explaining. None of these responses are consciously chosen by the individual, but every one of us has an automatic tendency towards one.

Fawning in particular is often associated with childhood trauma, as a way of trying to avoid abuse through placating the abuser in a pre-emptive move. Extreme people-pleasers who are afraid to say what they think and always put themselves above others will often have learnt this behaviour as a method of ensuring their own safety.

Imagine someone standing over you and shouting at you loudly. They are intimidating and invading your personal space. How do you respond?

Fight, flight, freeze or fawn			
Fight	Flight	Freeze	Fawn
Clenched fists	Desire to hide	Difficulty	People
Fast heart rate	or run away	speaking	pleasing
Arguing	Feeling	Shutting down	Great
Shouting	trapped	Desire to hide	difficulty
Desire	Wide eyes	Trembling or	saying 'no'
to punch	Anxiety	shaking	Over-
something			apologising

How stress responses link to food

I have found in my clinical practice (and please note that these are only my own observations), that those who gravitate towards flight are especially inclined to use food as a coping mechanism. Food is an effective distraction and avoidance technique that helps the brain run away from its problems. Those who fawn may also gravitate towards food to soothe themselves and establish some sense of self again following the loss of identity that can accompany fawning. I find those who freeze tend towards an avoidance of food to cope. Those who fight may end up turning to food as a result of shame experienced after the event, which we will explore later.

Not everyone who experiences trauma turns to food, and not everyone who has a disordered relationship with food has experienced trauma. We all have a stress response that has a tendency towards one of these four, and we all have a window of tolerance that we need tools to cope with when we are overwhelmed.

With all this in mind, I offer you the following questions:

- Are there events in my life that I could describe as traumatic?
- Have I processed these experiences for what they are?
- What is my core belief about myself?
- What does my window of tolerance look like?
- Do I have a tendency towards fight, flight, freeze or fawn?

If, having read this, you are concerned that you have experienced trauma that you have not yet processed, and you are relying on food to cope with this, please know that you are not alone and you do not have to suffer in silence. It can be tempting to immediately want to rush into doing something with this, but I encourage you to pause and sit with it. Then, at the end of this book, you'll find some information about seeking therapeutic support that can help you process your experiences. In the meantime, let's continue exploring.

3

Food and Love

'Food can never leave me like he did.'

Several years ago, Jemima was dumped by her long-term boyfriend. It left her absolutely heartbroken. Since then she had tried to date several times. She tried creating a dating profile but would stop herself every time and instead choose to go on a diet. She felt that she could only date once she had lost weight. It would take several months of work with me before she recognised that this was simply an excuse and a cover for her poor self-worth. There is no judgement in my use of the word 'excuse' here – all brains use comfortable cover narratives all the time, as they enable us to live in denial. Cover narratives mean that we don't have to think about the deeper concern at play. For someone who doesn't believe that they hold a lot of worth, it is far more comfortable to focus on the process and journey of dieting than it is to examine how they feel about themselves. Dieting is a far more comfortable process to focus on than self-worth.

Most people I meet are unhappy with themselves regardless of their body size. The number of times I've had people describe how unhappy they are with their bodies is too great to count. They attribute their unhappiness to their size, only to then remember that when they were thinner they were also not happy. But this uncomfortable truth often gets denied. It might sound hard to believe, but it's not about the end goal of being thin: the diet itself, and the focus on weight loss, is a diversion from the real issue at hand. The process is the distraction. The goal is simply what is dictated by society. If we're focused on dieting, it leaves very little headspace to examine our relationship with ourselves, to consider that deep down we might not feel that we're good enough or worthy of being loved.

The lie that thinness creates happiness plays a significant role in this. Now, there's no denying that when you are in a smaller body the world treats you better. You can fit into plane seats, you can buy clothes in regular shops, you can go to your doctor and have your symptoms listened to rather than simply being asked if you'd considered Weight Watchers. Society benefits those who are thin. It's not designed to accommodate fat bodies. On the one hand, therefore, thinness can lead to greater satisfaction simply because others treat you better and you receive less judgement; however, it is not the complete picture. On the other hand, all the validation from the outside world can't heal your self-loathing, but that doesn't stop people from trying.

Losing weight instead of losing love

I have met plenty of people who would rather focus on losing weight than develop a close relationship with another human being, or attempt intimacy with a stranger, or find someone who loves us unconditionally. They would rather focus on their body than love. People can reject you – food can't. But you can reject food. This unequal relationship means that we feel we're in control and that we have power.

Food can feel like love. Food is there when people go away; food doesn't hurt you; food doesn't say you're not good enough; food tastes good; food always comforts. But food is only a substitute for love. When people binge or overeat, they reinforce the idea that people can't offer them what they need, whereas food can, so they give themselves food and their brain on some level feels that they are in control. Except that they're not really in control. Most people I speak to describe the urge to eat as not being a choice but more as something that overcomes them, an itch that is so intense it desperately needs to be scratched. But food begins as something to control when love from others cannot be controlled.

Our relationship with food is a microcosm of everything we have learned about loving and being loved, and what we deserve in life. It is the stage upon which we re-enact our relationships and our beliefs about ourselves. Unsurprisingly, the lessons we learn about love begin in early childhood, with our parents. Research shows that people who describe themselves as emotional eaters are more likely to report difficult childhood family relationships, including feeling lonely, a lack of connection, and a lack of self-care in adulthood.[9] When conditions are placed on the love our parents offer us, our attachments to food and other people become messy and insecure.

Attachment theory is a fascinating area of psychology. It suggests that the earliest relationships we have in life, usually with parents or caregivers, shape us significantly in our relationships with others throughout our life, which, as we have seen, can impact our relationship with food.

Psychologist John Bowlby described attachment as a lasting psychological connectedness between human beings. He was the first significant researcher in this area and was curious to understand the separation anxiety that children experience when they're separated from their primary caregivers. He believed that the earliest bonds formed between children and caregivers ripple across our entire lives. He posited that if primary caregivers are available and responsive to a child's needs, it enables the child to develop a sense of security, which gives them a solid foundation on which to explore the world. But what happens when our parents or caregivers are not available and not responsive to our needs?

In the 1970s, psychologist Mary Ainsworth performed a ground-breaking experiment called the Strange Situation. She observed children between the ages of twelve months and eighteen months as they responded to a situation where they were left alone and then reunited with a caregiver. Based on this, Mary Ainsworth described three styles of attachment: secure, anxious insecure and avoidant insecure. A fourth was later added by other researchers: anxious avoidant.

Anxious attachment is characterised by just that: anxiety. When a parent leaves, there is great distress and children learn that their parents are not available or to be depended upon. Those with anxious attachment styles often grow up to be incredibly hyper-aware of their partner's feelings, with a constant fear that they will leave.

Avoidant attachment involves avoidance. Children tend to not be too fussed when their parents leave, usually because of a sense of punishment when relying on a caregiver. This often occurs as a result of abusive or neglectful parents. In adulthood, those with avoidant-attachment styles tend to distance themselves from partners, find difficulty in asking for help, and are more likely to withdraw if something is wrong.

Children who grow up with secure attachments are more likely to have strong romantic relationships simply because they start with the belief that they are worthy, that other people are dependable and available, and that you can trust them.

Some people believe that attachment styles cannot be changed. I don't believe that to be true. I firmly believe that people are able to learn a secure attachment style. This can be through a therapist who is reliable and available (but with good boundaries) or through a romantic relationship with a partner who is securely attached. But although attachment styles can improve, they can also change for the worse in adulthood. Having a traumatic experience in a romantic relationship, whether that is abuse, rape or rejection, can foster anxious or avoidant attachment styles, either through an anxiety that everyone will leave you, by sabotaging any relationship that begins to get serious, or through avoiding relationships completely out of fear of repeating the same pattern. For this reason, I want to explore food and love both in childhood and in adulthood.

Food love is learned

Our behaviours around food don't just come out of nowhere. No one suddenly wakes up one day and decides to starve themselves or decides to eat a pizza and a tub of ice cream and a box of cookies and a loaf of garlic bread. These things don't happen for no reason. For some of us it comes from our relationships with others, for some it stems from not learning that we are lovable in childhood, for others it comes from losing the belief that we are lovable in adulthood.

A child who has been abused will tend to believe that it is their fault, and an adult who binge eats will tend to believe that they have no self-control. Now, instead of getting angry at an abuser, that person can direct their anger inward towards themselves. As Geneen Roth, bestselling author of *When Food is Love*, writes, 'Diets and food plans enable adults to remain children, victims of oppressive familial and cultural systems in which they spend their lives punishing themselves for not being good enough.'

For some people, they learned that food is love, and therefore depriving themselves of food is an effective form of punishment when they feel they don't deserve to show themselves love. For others, their parents were absent, abusive or inconsistent, and food was there as a comforting warm blanket of love when people weren't. They may also use food as punishment because they don't think they deserve better. When we haven't been loved well, we stop expecting that others will fulfil our needs and instead learn to rely only on ourselves. And so we eat.

For some people, the connection between food and love is incredibly explicit. They learned that the love from their parents is conditional on their body looking a certain way, so if they gain weight, they are no longer loved, they are no longer good enough and must change in order to receive love again. For these people, going on a diet, becoming smaller, or eating less food can be ways of trying to be worthy of love from others.

When Tolu's parents got divorced, her mother used to comfort eat in order to cope. Whenever she did this, she encouraged Tolu to join in. It was their way of bonding and supporting each other during this difficult time. Every time she diets, it makes her think of her father, who she does not get on with, which results in the diet being unsustainable. Instead, she comfort eats to bring herself closer to her mother again. This was an unconscious process for her before we made it conscious.

Xena was constantly criticised and overlooked by her mother, and she described her mother to me as overbearing and suffocating. Food was just one arena of many where this would play out. At the dinner table, her brothers would receive as much food as they wanted while her plate was constantly scrutinised just in case she ate too much. Her mother's love was conditional upon her eating the right amount of food: not so little that it was perceived to be a rejection of her cooking, not so much that it would warrant criticism and fear of weight gain. She started secret eating at night to find comfort and love in the food she was denied.

It is not always clear why people turn to food instead of other options. One reason is that there is such a clear connection between food and the body. Another is that food is the first source of comfort and also the first opportunity for rebellion we have in life. What do I mean by this? In an ideal environment, our very first experience of eating is associated with the comfort of being held in a caregiver's arms. As a baby, our life is largely dictated by our parents. Children only have two main opportunities to exert power: one is to reject food, the other is to excrete it. Food in and food out. Substances like drugs and alcohol don't always hold that level of significance in people's lives (unless there's a family history, of course). Food, on the other hand, does for every single one of us.

Security and food

When our attachment style is insecure, food can become a secure attachment. That's why it's so hard to let it go even when we feel it no longer serves us. If, after reading this chapter, you've identified that your attachment style is likely insecure, you can now work with this knowledge and awareness. After all, before we decide where we want to go, we have to know where we are. You may now feel able to start recognising certain behaviours or thoughts you have around dating and romantic relationships as part of your attachment style.

- Are you telling yourself that you can't date until you go on a diet?
- Do you find yourself engaging in emotional eating when a date goes badly?
- Do you find yourself eating in response to rejection?
- Do you deny yourself food as a form of punishment after an argument with someone?
- If you're anxiously attached, does being in a relationship with an avoidant person drive you to eat more?
- If you have an avoidant attachment style, does being in a relationship with an anxious person drive you to eat differently?

For as long as you are fixated on your weight as the problem, you have an excuse not to be physically intimate with someone, or even go on a date. It's not actually about losing weight, because once that armour is no longer preventing closeness with another person, there's no excuse left, and that in itself is terrifying to the point where another excuse has to be found ('I'm too busy, I have too much work to do, it's not the right time', and so on). If this sounds like you, I wonder what you are really frightened of. What were your early life experiences of love and being loved? Did something happen that has made you afraid of intimacy and being loved? To quote Geneen Roth, 'We become frightened of intimacy because our intimate experiences were frightening, not because we are incapable of loving. If we are ever to deeply love ourselves – or anyone else – we must first examine why we are frightened.'

Perhaps it's time to stop making excuses and find out what's really going on underneath. These questions I've posed can guide you, and that knowledge can drive you forward towards change. As someone who has navigated the transition from an anxious attachment style to a secure one, 1 know it's possible with deep self-exploration and a supportive guide.

Many of my clients have expressed their frustration to me that people around them just don't understand. They don't understand when they don't want to go to see their parents for Christmas or go on a blind date. When you had a happy childhood, you assume everybody else has too. Not everyone gets to experience unconditional love from their parents. Not everybody has a secure attachment growing up.

4

Parents and Emotions

Childhood is an incredibly important time for our self-development and our brain development. We are like sponges absorbing information in any form that is offered. All this information, these messages, these lessons shaped the way that we see the world and the way that we see ourselves as adults. But that does not mean that these messages are always helpful, especially when it comes to our relationship with our emotions.

In many families, emotions are simply not discussed openly. They may be felt or implied, but kept hidden. If you have been taught that emotions such as sadness, loneliness, fear, anger or jealousy are bad emotions that you need to avoid, you will do whatever it takes to suppress them. The thing is, you are human; therefore you will feel all these feelings at some point, so here is my question to you: how do you deal with these feelings when you've never been taught how? One way is with food.

We learn from others

'Boys don't cry.'
    'Don't get angry, you know I hate it.'

'Stop crying or I'll give you something to cry about.'

The above statements are obvious examples of emotional suppression. They very explicitly tell someone not to feel what they're feeling, or not to express that emotion. But these messages can also be incredibly subtle and heavily implied. In my experience, that does not make the messages any less powerful or impactful. Modelling is a key method through which we learn from others: by mimicking what they do. If our parents don't cry in front of us and react awkwardly when we cry, this may teach us that this is not acceptable. It says, 'that's just not something we do here'. If you could see that a parent was upset, and they absolutely insisted they were OK, or if they are adamant that 'I'm not angry, I'm just disappointed', despite exhibiting very clear signs of anger, this can also lead to confusion around emotions. If parents push a strong solution-focused approach on to their children that doesn't allow for time and space to feel first, it might send the message that emotions are there to be solved, not felt. Don't get me wrong, solutions are great, but emotions need to be felt first, and what happens when that child is placed in a situation where there is no immediate solution to be found? They struggle to cope.

The opposite can also be true: if emotions are completely unchecked and uncontained, that can also teach us that these emotions are bad and should be avoided; for example, Hazel had a brother who would regularly fly into fits of rage at the smallest thing. His anger was totally uncontained and intense to witness. From this, Hazel learned to tread carefully around other people's anger and not to add to the burden of others by bringing her own anger into the midst. Now she has a real inability to feel and express any kind of anger, choosing instead to turn to food to push the anger down again. This serves two purposes: firstly, it nicely suppresses the feelings of anger; secondly, it redirects it towards the self rather than a situation or another person, as now she can feel angry at herself for having 'eaten too much'. When someone has experienced rage and violence as a result of anger, it is perhaps not surprising that there is a degree of unacceptability that lingers around anger, and a deep fear of becoming just like the person who rages. That fear is incredibly powerful.

When parents are uncontained with their emotions, it teaches children to tiptoe around them. These children grow up far too quickly. They become the caregivers of their parents' emotions. They learn to anticipate and notice the subtlest of hints in others that might offer them a clue as to how they are feeling. Ethan's father was an alcoholic. He learned from a young age to be hypervigilant around him, noticing exactly how he opened the door and entered the house after work. Through this Ethan established some sense of control at identifying which father was coming home each day; would it be the sober father who was critical but fairly benign? Or would it be the drunk father who was hurtful, neglectful and angry? Through experiences like this, children learn to put others' emotional needs above their own for their own sense of safety. It is their way of staying alive. While Ethan was a child, this was his way of keeping safe – and it worked. It was incredibly effective. But that same need to put others first stuck around until his forties, long after he moved away from his father. It is no longer needed, but the brain takes a while to catch up with a sense of safety because moving those barriers, removing that wall, that defence mechanism, that protective factor, is a massive risk. It's understandable that the brain would be reluctant to get rid of something that once worked so well. But the reality is that for Ethan, continuing to put others first, even thirty years later, has been at the expense of his own happiness, and being so aware of other people's emotions led to him suppressing his own with food. It was time to let this go.

While someone is still living with their parents, I believe it is incredibly difficult for these safety mechanisms to change, arguably impossible, when we are still in the same situation and the same location that invited that safety mechanism in the first place and caused it to take root. There is no incentive for that to change; however, once we have some sense of independence and we are away from the people and situation that brought about this strategy, we can begin to unlearn and relearn the safety of a new environment.

Having said that, the process is not necessarily going to be an easy one. The messages we learned from our parents in early childhood are the blueprint on which we base our understanding of ourselves and the world. It's not easy to change a blueprint after the building is already constructed. It involves going right back to the foundations of our understanding of ourselves and laying new ground. It is so much more than simply changing a behaviour. This may sound incredibly pessimistic, but I believe that having a realistic understanding of what this work involves allows us to have compassion for ourselves when the going gets tough. Of course, it's tough. Changing a blueprint was never going to be easy. If it's easy, it's probably not a blueprint.

Understanding yourself without blame

I want to be very clear that none of this is about blame. I am not interested in playing a blame game with parents. It is dull and unhelpful. This is about understanding why you are the way you are. It's about being curious about yourself and where your ideas about yourself and the world may have come from. Of course, plenty of these will come from parents and caregivers, because in our first few years of life they are often the only consistent influence that we have. It is not our fault if we have internalised the negative messages that we were given as children. We do that because we are supposed to – that's how brains work. We arguably would have internalised them if they were positive too. If you're still feeling guilty, please remember that nobody has to know what you discover about yourself unless you choose to share it with them.

I want to repeat that: the messages you learned and internalised about yourself and your emotions are not your fault. You did not choose to learn them – you didn't have a choice. The family environment that you grew up in is your normal. It is not until later in life that we begin the process of comparison to others, and by then those messages and lessons have often taken root. We are not to blame as children because we didn't have the power to choose. It's not your fault, but it is your responsibility to do something about it when you become aware as an adult. You are no longer a helpless child, you are now an adult who can give yourself these supportive messages and lessons that you wish you'd been taught earlier. Of course, an effective therapist can be a huge help with this. Some people call this therapeutic work 'inner child work'. If the idea of opening up to your child-self feels a bit awkward or uncomfortable, try simply thinking about it as a process of self-discovery. You're not literally talking to yourself as a child, it's a metaphor for understanding yourself. If this concept does connect with you, this may be something that's worth exploring. Some people find it helpful to talk to the inner child as they would a living person. They find it helpful to ask them what they need, to validate their feelings, to tell them they are good enough. It is a way of re-parenting yourself, by offering yourself what your parents were unable or unwilling to give you, or simply didn't quite give you in the way that you needed.

The messages we receive from our parents are rarely intentionally harmful. Often parents pass messages along to us that they themselves received and perceived as either helpful or as simply the way things are done. They may have never questioned their relationship with emotions before. This message we receive could be as simple as being overly solution focused. We may be taught that focusing on solutions is of great benefit, and I agree that it can be, but not at the expense of actually feeling things. Too often I see people who have been brought up in a very solution-focused household bypass the feeling stage to go straight to the solution. This is what they were always encouraged to do. Why stand around wasting time feeling when you can simply solve the problem? This sounds incredibly efficient; however, my concern is that if the emotion doesn't have time to be recognised, sat with and discharged, have you really solved the problem? You may have solved what the emotion was triggered by, but that doesn't guarantee that the emotion will disappear. In fact, it might just push it down, only for it to resurface later. Again, I notice this often with feelings such as anger, sadness and jealousy. If I am angry and I diffuse the situation or walk away, the problem is solved, so then why am I walking towards the nearest restaurant and placing an order without even thinking about it? If I feel sad, but I then tell myself what's the point in feeling sad as I can't change anything, does that make the sadness go away, or do I now simply feel frustrated with myself for feeling sad? If I feel jealous because someone has something I want and I simply throw money at the problem, does that really meet my needs? Sometimes, yes; but not always.

Slowly releasing emotions

Our emotions are stored in our bodies, and when we ignore them and push them down they will eventually resurface in ways that we can't necessarily expect. Imagine a volcano bubbling away inside you. A surge of emotion causes the steam to rise, but then instead of letting it out you place a giant stopper on the main vent. Problem solved. Well, not really. Allow enough pressure to build up in this confined space and suddenly it becomes too much. Now, instead of exploding upwards in a predictable manner, all that pressure is released without warning through a side vent you didn't even know existed. Suddenly you're having to do damage control while also trying to figure out what the hell just happened. If you have ever exploded at someone for a minor inconvenience, or suddenly started crying because one minor incident went wrong, you may have some idea of what I'm referring to. We don't have to push those emotions down. If we allow the pressure to be slowly released in a contained and gradual manner over the course of days and weeks, we cannot completely prevent an explosion but we can drastically reduce the risk. That sounds much healthier to me. I understand that this can be incredibly intimidating if you've been taught that these emotions are wrong, if you've been taught these emotions should be avoided, or if your experience says these emotions are dangerous. Just because an emotion is unacceptable or dangerous in somebody else does not mean that it has to be in you. Just because somebody you grew up with had volatile bursts of rage does not mean that you will be the same. You are not that person. It's time to allow yourself to simply be you.

With that in mind, here are some questions you may want to answer for yourself:

- What did I learn about emotions as a child?
- How did significant adults in my life (parents, caregivers, teachers) respond to my emotions?
- How did people react when I felt sad and cried?
- How was anger expressed when I was growing up?
- How do I feel about crying in front of others?
- How do I feel about being honest with others about how I am feeling?

5

Diet Culture

We are all born into diet culture. From a young age we are taught that certain bodies are better than others. Thin bodies are good bodies, while fat bodies are bad bodies. If you are thin, you are praised by society, you are valued, you are seen as good, efficient, disciplined, neat and having willpower. If you're in a larger body, you are seen as lazy, greedy, undesirable, undisciplined, unmotivated. In a nutshell: not good enough.

Food and bodies are so interconnected because the food we eat becomes our body. That is unavoidable. There is such a strong overlap of disordered eating and body image issues that, in my experience, you rarely get one without the other. We see food as a way to manipulate, sculpt and control our bodies into the shape that we desire, or rather, that society tells us we should desire.

We have learned to associate aesthetic desirability with health and worth, such that the ideal standard of health is now the exact same as the ideal standard of beauty. The impacts of this are far reaching and terrifying to imagine. Rates of eating disorders have never been higher, while services are completely unable to keep up and are chronically underfunded. The exact figure varies, but a 2020 survey by the Women and Equalities

Committee show that 61 per cent of adults and 66 per cent of children in the UK feel negative towards their body.[10] That means most of us are unhappy with our bodies, and when people dislike their body, they will engage in all sorts of deeply unhealthy behaviours in order to achieve what is seen as a healthy body. By trying to pursue health, we are engaging in behaviours that are unhealthy. Where on Earth is the sense in that?

There's a lot to unpack here. It's hard to know where to begin, but let's start with the obvious route that many people take, which is dieting to lose weight.

More complex than weight

Much of what we have been told about health and weight is an oversimplification. BMI, or body mass index, was created as a population-based tool and it is useful for the most part on large groups of people. However, although it is a crude method that doesn't accurately measure an individual's health, we rely on it because it is simple, easy to measure, doesn't require complex equipment and it correlates with health at the extreme ends of the spectrum. But using a single number to define health is never a good idea. Humans are incredibly complex, bodies are incredibly complex and so much more than just a single number. Imagine if we determined someone's health purely based on their blood pressure alone. I think it's safe to say that we'd be missing out on a lot of useful data. We would be incorrectly deeming people unhealthy due to white coat syndrome, a phenomenon where people's blood pressure increases simply because they feel nervous about going to see a doctor. We would be accidentally categorising people as healthy when their blood pressure is low, even though other biomarkers such as blood sugar levels, for example, might be high and therefore putting them at risk of type-2 diabetes. Imagine going to the doctor with a legitimate concern around abdominal pain only for them to immediately test your blood pressure and make the entire conversation about reducing it, when that has nothing to do with your initial concern in the first place. Sounds frustrating, doesn't it? Conversations like this happen all the time. I know, because people tell me about them. I know, because people in larger bodies go to see their doctor far less frequently out of fear of being dismissed, which results in serious concerns being overlooked and progressing further before being caught and treated.

Of course, not all healthcare professionals treat people like this, but there are enough that we have a serious problem. Weight bias has been documented in dietitians, doctors, nurses and psychologists; for example, psychologists will say that a fat patient has more severe symptoms and a worse prognosis compared with when a patient is thin, even if they present with identical psychological profiles.[11] In 2013, an assessment of trainee dietitians, doctors, nurses and nutritionists showed that 98 per cent had some degree of fatphobia and negative attitudes towards people in larger bodies.[12] That's an unacceptably high number.

I'm not going to sit here and tell you that there is absolutely zero relationship between weight and health. Of course there is a link with certain health conditions. If we go back to the blood pressure example, there are situations where having high blood pressure is genuinely hypertension and increases the risk of heart disease and stroke considerably. But the assumption that everyone who is above a certain BMI is unhealthy and that everyone below a certain BMI is healthy is incredibly damaging. If you had to guess which BMI category is associated with the lowest risk of early death, you'd probably say the 'normal' category of BMl, which is between 18.5 and 25. You would be wrong. The BMl category with the lowest risk of early death according to millions of data points is in fact the 'overweight' category.[13] In the elderly population, those who are 'overweight' actually live longer than their lighter counterparts.[14] so when we tell patients who are in the 'overweight' category to lose weight, are we in fact potentially causing harm?

The diet business

Diets are an incredibly successful business model based on finding repeat customers. The more people try and fail diets, the more these companies gain profit. If there was actually one single diet that was incredibly effective above everything else, everyone would do it, lose weight, and the whole industry would shut down. But that's not what happens. The majority of people who go on a diet stick with it, lose some weight, and after a year they struggle to maintain it. Research shows that between one-third and two-thirds of weight is regained within one year and almost all is regained within five years.[15] Other research says that after two years, individuals who report trying to diet end up at a higher weight than before.[16] Some people are incredibly successful on diets long term. They manage to lose weight and maintain that weight loss over many years, but these people are very clearly the minority. Why, then, do the majority of people find that they're unable to lose weight successfully while dieting long term? Some prominent and loud voices attribute this to the fact that we live in an environment that makes it very easy for people who don't have willpower to keep eating and gaining weight. Others keep it even simpler and say, well, people simply don't have willpower. I have a much more nuanced and optimistic view of humanity.

A global survey carried out across thirty countries in 2020 found that 45 per cent of people said they are currently trying to lose weight.[17] Of these, most are trying to reduce their sugar intake or their overall calorie intake. Slightly older research from 2016 focusing on the UK shows that half of Brits have tried to lose weight, and that most of those are trying to be on a diet all or most of the time.[18]

How your body reacts to dieting

Is it really reasonable to suggest that half the population doesn't have any willpower? That they are failing at dieting because they just can't maintain it due to a lack of motivation and inner strength? That doesn't sound right to me. The way I see it, there are a number of reasons why it's so difficult to lose weight and then maintain that weight loss. Firstly, we have basic evolutionary biology, which shows your body doesn't like you losing weight. Many generations ago, humans lived in an environment where food was not always around and there were times of feast and times of famine. It makes sense, therefore, that the body would put on weight relatively quickly in times of feast and lose weight slowly in times of famine. Your body does this by slowing down your metabolism, discouraging you from moving as much so you don't expend as much energy, and helping you to conserve existing energy stores in your body. Your body can't tell the difference between being in an environment of starvation and voluntarily going on a diet. Intention doesn't really mean much here. This is why people on diets often feel very tired, understandably, as they're not getting enough energy to sustain their daily needs. This leads people to find it really difficult to move as much as they would normally do. Alongside this decrease in movement, hunger hormones are increased, thereby encouraging them to eat more. Research confirms this:[19] rigid dieting is usually broken up by periods of overeating, even in the absence of hunger.[20] In other words, you diet, then you overeat, then you beat yourself up about it and you restrict and diet again. Rinse and repeat.

Another reason why dieting is so hard is due to our psychology. As soon as you tell yourself that you can't have something, you push it to the forefront of your mind and now you're thinking about something that you weren't before and, oh boy, now you want it even more. This is why tobacco companies are big fans of no smoking signs, and why if I ask you not to think about puppies you're now thinking about puppies. If you repeatedly tell yourself 'I can't eat chocolate', then your brain hears the words 'eat chocolate'. Now you're thinking about chocolate. In fact, I'm thinking about chocolate right now. I wasn't thinking about chocolate before I wrote this; it wasn't even in my mind at all. If it was there, it was lurking at the back completely out of my conscious thought process. But now it's there and I'm thinking about what chocolate I have in the house; I'm ranking the chocolate that I have from best to worst flavour-wise. I'm not even hungry right now! This isn't a matter of willpower. This is simply the way our brain functions.

The modern food environment

On top of all this, we have to add our current food environment, which is very different from our ancestral food environment. Many of us are in a position of great privilege where we don't have to think about where our next meal is coming from, and we have access to food almost 24/7. We are around food all the time, and not just any food, seriously delicious food too. We have food delivery apps, we can order groceries online and have them arrive within half an hour, we have recipe boxes that pre-measure all the ingredients for you. We can access food based on an immediate reaction rather than through careful consideration of what to cook.

Take all these reasons why dieting is so unsuccessful for so many people, add in a societal narrative that being fat is the worst thing you can be, and you have a recipe for psychological disaster.

I've focused on adults so far, but diet culture can affect us right through childhood as well. Children whose parents put them on diets are more likely to eat when not hungry and be overweight later in life,[21] which just shows how clearly dieting has the opposite effect to the one intended. Adolescents who are teased about their weight show higher levels of unhealthy food behaviours, such as starving themselves, purging or binge eating.[22] This is true whether those comments come from family or friends or bullies. Whether from children or adults, shaming people or making fun of them doesn't tend to inspire them to lose weight. In fact, it usually leads to weight gain.[23] The research consistently shows that people who are shamed and laughed at for their weight are less likely to engage in health-promoting behaviours. When you think about it, this makes sense. If you've been taught to feel shit about your body and that you should feel ashamed of it, it doesn't generally push you in the direction of wanting to take good care of yourself and give your body the nutrients it needs to thrive. Shaming doesn't help.

In my clinical experience, I find that a question that tends to bring out a lot of people's food and body stories is this: what did you learn about your body as a child? People will tell me stories of being taken to healthcare professionals as a child where they are poked and prodded and spoken about by strangers with no warning and no explanation. Of being told to strip, put on a gown and step on scales while a strange man in a white coat watches closely and tells their mother everything that's wrong with them. They speak of these ordeals with the terror of a confused child. Then they go home and suddenly they're eating different foods from their siblings. Some are explicitly told by their parents that they are too big and need to go on a diet. Others are simply told this change in diet is to make them healthier. For many, these strong memories have stayed with them all the way into late adulthood.

When did you first learn that your body was wrong? That it was too big? That it was unacceptable? Where did you learn that the kindness of others is dependent on your body size? The pain of learning this in childhood stays with people. It cuts deep into their very core and tells them that they're not good enough. These people often have a lifetime of dieting ahead of them. In my experience, it's only when they themselves have children and their children approach that same age that they were when they went on their first diet, that's when the panic sets in. It's like they see their whole dieting history flash before their eyes, and suddenly they worry that their children will follow the same path that they did. Only then, when it becomes about their child, are they able to acknowledge for themselves how painful, how fruitless, how thankless, how never-ending this task has been of trying to be good enough through changing their body. Suddenly they are exhausted and have had enough.

If the world tells you that your body is not good enough, that it makes you ugly and lazy, then of course you will do whatever it takes to change that. The answer to your problem is presented all around you: go on a diet. Look at all these success stories from people just like you! But then your story is not a success, not long-term anyway, so you try again and again and again, but it still doesn't last, and you are left with this feeling that you are unworthy. That is a shitty thing to learn. It is wrong. A person's worth is not tied to their weight. A person has intrinsic value no matter what.

I'm not here to tell you what to do. If you want to go on a diet, if you want to try to lose weight, if you want to change your body, by all means go ahead. Your body, your choice. That's how it should be. But I encourage you to just take a moment to consider: what are your reasons for going on a diet? We take it as a given that going on a diet and focusing on weight loss is the best option to improve health, but that's not the case for so many people. What is it that you're actually trying to achieve? When we take away the assumption that fat = bad and that dieting = health, what other options does this open up for you?

It's time to get curious about alternatives to dieting. Ask yourself:

- What would it be like to stop the dieting cycle?
- What would it be like to see your body as inherently having worth no matter its shape or size?
- What would it be like to treat yourself from a position of self-care rather than self-punishment?
- What would it mean to give yourself what your body needs rather than denying it and restricting it?

If you've reached this point in your life and you're fed up with dieting and fed up with feeling like your body is something to despise and not take care of, then you are welcome here. I have met so many people like you. You are not alone. I don't have to know you to be able to say that your worth is not dependent on being a certain size. I don't have to meet you to know that you have inherent worth and value no matter what you look like. You are good enough. You may not believe it right now, but you can learn to believe it. I've seen it happen over and over again, and it is a truly wonderful thing.

6

Shame

Shame is a sneaky little bastard. It worms its way into your brain and tells you that you are a bad person. Whereas guilt might have some productive purpose in many situations, shame rarely does. Guilt says 'I did a bad thing' – it's focused on the action. Shame says 'I am a bad person' – it's based on identity. It goes beyond the action to your fundamental core as a human being.

Researcher and author Brené Brown defines shame as, 'an intensely painful feeling or experience that we are flawed and therefore unworthy of love and belonging'. Shame can feel like a stone in the pit of our stomach, or a fog covering our entire body, or a rising heat that begins in the gut and ends in the face. We may avoid eye contact, hang our heads, make ourselves small. Shame can physically hurt.

Several conditions have to come together for someone to feel shame. Firstly, we have to be aware that we have transgressed some sort of norm. We must also perceive this norm as desirable and important. The final piece is the judgement of somebody, who can either be present or imagined.

Shame is not inherently bad, but both too much and too little can be harmful to us. Having no guilt or shame usually means you act inconsiderately. One of the reasons you don't take your shoes and socks off in an aeroplane is due to a fear of being publicly shamed by the other passengers. This is a good thing. Most people who come my way, however, have experienced too much shame, and it holds great power over them.

Secret eating

When it comes to food, shame drives people into secrecy. Shame says that your eating behaviour makes you a bad person, an unworthy person, and you can't possibly tell anybody about what's going on because they will judge you. Even when logically and rationally we know the people around us will offer us compassion and understanding, that niggling feeling of shame still lingers. The fear of judgement and shame is so powerful that it tends to override any rational argument.

In many ways I see secret eating as being similar to an affair. Psychotherapist and relationship expert Esther Perel writes brilliantly on the appeal of affairs. She describes how the appeal lies in the secrecy, that there is something rebellious and exciting about the forbidden nature of an affair. But once the affair is exposed and the couple are allowed to be together publicly, the appeal is lost. Many couples drift apart at this point as their relationship is no longer adrenaline fuelled. It feels dull and mundane in comparison. It loses all of its allure. Secret eating is quite similar in this way, but, rather than lust, the shame drives the secrecy, and the secrecy drives the shame. Once it's out in the open and we receive compassion and understanding from others instead of judgement, the anticipation and rebellion is also lost. It's not such a big deal anymore, and so the eating often decreases, because the shame spiral is broken.

Lola was a college student who was living with her parents to minimise her student debt. She came to see me because she found herself eating in secret whenever her parents were working. She would come home from college, check to see if anyone else was home, and raid the fridge. She expressed frustration because she couldn't understand why this was happening, as she wasn't eating due to hunger. To try to cope with this, she would aim to restrict all day, and found herself overeating even more when she came home. But only if there was no one home. If her parents were home and in the kitchen she would simply grab a snack and that would be it. It just so happens that Lola also used to eat in secret after school as a child to avoid judgement from her parents. As we started to draw the parallels between these two experiences – in her childhood when she went to school, and in her adulthood going to college – she started to understand what was happening and stopped judging herself so harshly. In both instances, she was returning home from education to a home she shared with her parents and eating in secret to avoid their judgement. Once she started working and moved out, the majority of her secret eating disappeared, because the shame and fear of judgement did.

The connection between shame and food goes beyond the obvious. When I first met Pietro he would regularly overeat. It would occur several times a week and only when he was alone. Whenever he was around others, his eating was arguably normal, in the sense that there was no under- or overeating. He simply ate until he felt full, enjoyed himself, and that was it. Something about being alone with his thoughts and his feelings was too difficult, however, and led him to turn to food. When we explored his life so far, he mentioned that he realised he was gay at a relatively young age. He came out to his parents and all was well, then he came out to his friends and they accepted him. Despite this, he is afraid of dating. He said, 'I've already been enough of a burden on my parents. I don't need to bring a partner home as well.' Considering the positive experience he had described when he came out to them, this surprised me. There was a contradiction there, and in my experience bringing this to the surface to explore usually leads to interesting insights. In Pietro's case, although his closest family and friends around him were very accepting of him, he was not accepting of himself. He felt his sexuality was a burden on those around him. He was, as he described it, OK with being gay in theory, but bringing a partner to meet friends and family would make it real. He was ashamed of that part of himself and who he loved. In our time together we named this as internalised homophobia. Despite all the progress we've made in society, there are still many messages that say if you deviate from the 'default' of heterosexual, there is something wrong with you. Many LGBTQ+ kids grow up feeling that they're not normal and their desires are something to be ashamed of.

The external manifestation of an internal struggle

There is a documented link between internalised homophobia, body image issues, and binge eating.[24] The body is the thing that does the desiring, and what it desires is deemed wrong, therefore the body is wrong. Because of the fear of judgement, there is secrecy, and the secrecy drives shame. When this is manifested in the body it can lead to binge eating, or a form of emotional eating that is driven by a sense of punishing the body for not being good enough, not 'correct', or for desiring the wrong thing. What outwardly presents as emotional eating is, at its core, an inability to accept the self. This, like so many things, is learned. No one is born feeling that they're not good enough. No one is born feeling wrong. But somewhere along the way we internalise these ideas if we are exposed to them.

Any kind of shame and -isms can be externalised to the body.

It feels easier to deal with because the body can be changed. We see the body as something we can control and food as a means of doing that, and so what starts as shame continues as hatred and punishment directed at our body. Food simply becomes the means of doing that. Then, after eating, there are more feelings of shame and guilt, and the self-critical voice (which I explain in detail later) kicks in. This only drives the cycle further. For some, this leads to drastic measures to compensate for their transgressions, like purging, restricting or over-exercise.

This is why a negative body image is often defined as an external manifestation of an internal struggle. It's much more comfortable to focus on the body. It's much more socially acceptable to say, 'I want to change my body' (external) rather than 'I feel that I'm wrong as a person' (internal). Often our inability to accept ourselves doesn't sit well with our progressive views on subjects such as sexuality. This cognitive dissonance, where we hold two conflicting beliefs at the same time, feels jarring, and we try to solve that in a way that makes it make sense for us. The body is an easy thing to focus on – not only is it deemed socially acceptable to dislike your body and to want to change it, but it's also often the first thing people notice about you. It's an obvious target. When you focus on your body, your brain feels calmer because it thinks it's solving the problem. Except it's not, not in the long term. Long term, self-acceptance is the answer.

A learned behaviour

Shame is learned. We learn it from the way people we love treat others, the way they treat themselves and the way they treat us. In extreme cases, this occurs when abusers blame their victims for their actions towards them. If this occurs to us at a young age, we may internalise the idea that we are to blame for what happens to us. Regardless, in abusive situations, shame and self-blame is often a survival mechanism, as standing up for yourself can be met with harsh punishment. We feel that there must be something inherently wrong and bad about us to be treated this way. This can then lead to feelings that we deserve what happened to us and we deserve to feel ashamed for being who we are. It also leads us to believe that we can't trust ourselves, which often drives the cycle of abuse. Early shame experiences can become embedded as part of our identity, leading us to believe that others will not accept us, and that we are not worthy of love and connection. In less extreme scenarios, we can still learn from our primary caregivers that we should feel ashamed of who we are. Even if that is not their intention, if we are dismissed, if our emotions and concerns are not taken seriously, if our parents put us on a well-intentioned diet, if we hear our family make derogatory comments about others' bodies, we may still internalise the idea that we are not good enough and feel shame.

As I said before, I'm not here to play the blame game. As humans we tend to judge and shame others in areas where we ourselves feel vulnerable to shame. It distracts from ourselves and places the focus on someone else; for example, those who will fat-shame others usually have the strongest internalised fatphobia. Those who shame others for the way they eat usually have the greatest insecurity around food themselves. People who have a good relationship with food don't judge others for what they eat because they recognise that it's absolutely none of their business. Yes, some of us use shame because we want others to do better. We think it's an effective tool for change, even though the research consistently says that it isn't; however, a lot of shame comes from a place of insecurity.

Considering how the majority of people feel insecure about

their body, it's not surprising that bodily shame is a whole category unto itself. In fact, it is so common that there are two
types of bodily shame. 'Current bodily shame' is experienced in
relation to our current body size, whereas 'anticipated bodily
shame' occurs in relation to the anticipation of shame if we were
to gain weight. In other words, it has the ability to affect anyone
of any size. You can thank societal fatphobia for that one.

Brené Brown says, 'Shame drives two big tapes, "never good
enough", and, if you can talk it out of that one, "who do you
think you are?".' I hear this in the way people say to me:

'I shouldn't feel so anxious around food'.

'This shouldn't be so hard. I should be able to do this.'

'It's my fault I'm fat.'

'I'm so embarrassed I can't just get it together and eat
normally.'

'I can't tell people what's going on; they'll look at me
differently.'

I have seen too many people feel ashamed and embarrassed
around their food and eating behaviours. I have sat with people
crying tears of shame at having eaten due to stress the night
before. I've witnessed the frustration of people feeling ashamed
for not being able to eat enough to gain weight during eating
disorder recovery. I have heard the most intelligent people I
know call themselves an idiot for not being able to eat 'normally'. I have listened to too many people blame themselves for
things that are not even remotely their fault. I understand why
they feel that way. They say, 'people just don't understand'. And
they're right. If you barely think about food – if you don't know
what it's like to have disordered eating – of course you have no
idea. Unfortunately, that lack of understanding leads to dis-
missive comments, exasperated sighs and unhelpful judgements
that drive shame further.

I hold such a deep admiration for all those who are open with me about their shame. Shame is hard to discuss, and when we do touch it, our instinct is to quickly move to cover ourselves up. Understandably, we then want to hide, get away from it or pretend it isn't there. To name it and confront it head on is perhaps one of the hardest things we can do in life. One of my clients described it to me as jumping out of an aeroplane without checking to see if you have a parachute.

The pain of shame

Shame can be painful and debilitating and leave us feeling worse about ourselves than before. Whereas guilt often allows room for improvement (especially once a genuine apology is made), shame usually simply makes way for self-criticism. It's no surprise, then, that shame is highly correlated with depression, anxiety, eating disorders, low self-esteem, aggression, and more. People who are shame-prone are much more likely to internalise perceived wrongdoing. Rather than thinking, 'I made a mistake, I feel bad, I'm going to apologise', their thoughts are focused on the self, 'I'm such an idiot, I can't get anything right.' Those who are shame prone will often craft a shame narrative about themselves and repeat this until they believe it fully. From then on, they examine all their experiences in life through the lens of not being good enough.

Shame mediates the depressive pathway to addiction, including alcohol misuse and gambling. It also drives binge eating in men and women. In fact, binge eating can be a way of attempting to cope with shame, either by suppressing and avoiding it (like with many other emotions), or by punishing ourselves for it. Shame leads to binge eating, which then leads to more shame and distress afterwards. Seeing as it's such a vicious cycle, why does it stick around? Why doesn't the brain see that this isn't working? We may have been taught from a young age that we need to beat ourselves up in order to make a positive change in our lives and be better. We may have been encouraged to do so by authority figures in our lives. We may even have been shamed by authority figures, whether that's parents, caregivers or teachers. If shame is part of our blueprint then we will keep coming back to it until we unlearn it. It doesn't work though – not in the long term. Instead, it simply leads to secrecy, fear, disconnection, dissatisfaction, unhappiness and a reinforcement that we're not good enough.

Shame occupies this dual space, where it presents as both a cause of disordered eating and a barrier that prevents us from change. Shame is paralysing. The fear of current and future shame, embarrassment and judgement is so powerful that it prevents us from working towards acceptance, compassion and looking after ourselves with more kindness. But the great thing about fear is that you can face it and walk straight through to the other side.

- What are you afraid will happen if you open up to someone about what you're ashamed of?
- What are you afraid will happen if you stop hating your body?
- What do you hope could happen?

PART III

BARRIERS

7

Defence Mechanisms

Freud has entered the chat.

Sigmund Freud gets a little bit of a bad rep. He's not very popular at the moment. Despite his eccentric habits and sometimes unusual view of the world, one thing he did nail (pun intended) was defence mechanisms, although he called them 'ego defences'. Later, his daughter, Anna Freud[25] elaborated on his ideas and developed the concept into the well-known phenomenon we use in casual conversation today.

Although there are many categorisations and types of defence mechanisms, I'm going to focus on the few that, in my experience, are most relevant to our relationship with food.

Denial

We all have defence mechanisms. They are there to try to protect us. The most obvious, and perhaps the most common defence mechanism is denial. If reality is too much to handle, denial helps us to block it out by refusing to acknowledge its existence. In everyday life, denial is actually incredibly helpful. If we take the Covid-19 pandemic as an example, being consciously aware of the risk of getting ill every minute of every day would keep us in a state of hyper awareness and arousal that would be too overwhelming and too much to deal with. We need to be in denial sometimes in order simply to get on with our day, get our work done, wash the dishes, make food, take care of ourselves or whatever we need. In this way, denial has its benefits. Of course, we can also easily use denial in our everyday lives to avoid dealing with painful feelings or areas of our life that we wish weren't happening. This can easily stray into the unhelpful or outright harmful. To continue with the example, being in denial about Covid while cooking or watching TV is arguably helpful. But dealing with denial while planning a gathering with friends during a pandemic is actively harmful.

If you are navigating a difficult relationship with food, denial can prevent you from seeking out the help and support that you need. It keeps you exactly where you are and helps you avoid change. I say 'helps' because the uncertainty of change is often frightening enough to keep us right where we're at. This is often one reason why many people stay in unhappy relationships, for example. The certainty of being miserable is preferable to the uncertainty of what lies ahead if they were to break up. We will often choose certain discomfort and pain over uncertainty.

If someone is in a state of denial around a coping mechanism they have in place to deal with their emotions – whether that is food or alcohol or drugs – they are unlikely to want to admit to it and seek help. Someone at this stage is unlikely to be willing to listen. As difficult as it is, sometimes we need to leave people there for a while. We cannot force people out of denial. Temporarily we sometimes can, but as soon as they are able to, people will slip right back into it. Denial can feel cosy, familiar and comforting in comparison to the unknown, or in comparison to what someone is trying to avoid.

Sometimes I find that people will come to clinic describing

unhappiness with their relationship with food. They will happily admit that their relationship with food is not what they want it to be and ask for my support in helping to get that to a better place. When confronted with the potential reasons why they eat, whether that be as a result of trauma, shame, diet culture or emotional suppression, there can be strong denial and an unwillingness to admit that there was a problem that needs solving, especially if it is something uncomfortable. I find that people infinitely prefer the narrative of 'I'm gaining weight, and therefore I have a problem', rather than examining the reasons why the weight gain is happening and why they are eating in this particular way. I understand why for many people it's much more comfortable to discuss their weight gain than it is to discuss their childhood trauma. The issue is that food is the solution, not the problem. But that's not necessarily what people want to hear.

Grief and denial

Denial is often considered the first stage of grief. In no particular order people cycle between denial, despair, bargaining and anger, hopefully reaching a place of acceptance. I've had my fair share of battles with avoidance and denial. The most powerful example I can share follows the death of my father. He died very suddenly: one day he was healthy and cycling 50 miles several times a week, the next day his heart stopped. He was fifty-eight. I was already in weekly therapy at this point in my life, and obviously much of our time was dedicated to this. A couple of weeks after his passing, my therapist asked me how I was feeling. I said I was actually doing OK. He looked me square in the eye and said, 'If you think you're OK, there's something very, very wrong.' Annoyingly, he was right. I had been avoiding going through the process of grief, because it was too painful and because I told myself that I had too much work to do. The narrative in my brain was that I didn't have the time to grieve. That was an excuse, of course – in reality I just didn't want to accept what had happened. My therapist gently encouraged me to set some time aside each day to process my grief. Reluctantly, I gave it a try and found myself crying every single day. I felt worse at first; I got angry at my therapist for making me do this. My brain started bargaining by showing me dreams where my father was still alive or by imagining scenarios where I could go back in time and save him. My despair was so intense that every time I cried I felt worse than before. My therapist allowed me to let all these feelings out and then some. Over time, through repeated conversation and repeated processing of my emotions, I found acceptance. This doesn't mean that I don't feel sad sometimes, and it doesn't mean that I don't miss him. It does mean that most of the time I can talk about what happened without feeling overwhelmed by my emotions. The process was painful and long, and so, so worth it.

While we associate grief with death, there are many more losses we can experience in life, such as the loss of the childhood we thought (or wish) we had. There can also be a loss of the 'good parent'. When someone has experienced abuse in childhood, they may label one of their parents the 'good parent' and the other as the 'bad parent'.* Roger had a father who was physically abusive, so he became the bad parent, while his mother became the good parent. During our time together he began to realise that his mother had been neglectful and, at times, cruel. His mother was unable to meet his needs and was

---

* This is actually a whole other process in psychodynamic psychotherapy known as 'splitting', which is where we divide people or things neatly into black and white, good and bad, as a coping mechanism.

unable to protect him from his father. He had to grieve the loss of the good parent he thought his mother was, in order to see the situation and his experiences accurately. Although this process was painful, it brought him closer to a place of acceptance and peace with his past.

That's the thing about denial and loss: at the end, the hopeful reward is acceptance. This is a beautiful and peaceful place where we can acknowledge the reality of our experiences without being overwhelmed by feelings of shame, discomfort, embarrassment, despair or anger.

Denial and acceptance

Many people I speak to have difficulty or uncertainty around this idea of acceptance. There are a number of misconceptions and assumptions attached to it that regularly come up.

For some, acceptance is misinterpreted as giving up or resignation, even though it is not these things. If you hold this assumption, you may want to try to note down the differences to disentangle these terms for yourself.

For some, denial is incredibly comfortable. The pain of acknowledging their experiences feels too much, the emotions attached to them too overwhelming, the memories just too many. Denial can feel like a peaceful bubble in comparison to facing our demons head on. But this bubble is an illusion that is keeping you trapped and small.

Others have a deeply held belief that they don't deserve to reach a place of freedom and acceptance because what happened to them is their fault. They blame themselves and therefore feel that they should suffer. As much as I can tell you this is untrue, you have to learn to believe it for yourself. Tell me: what is the appropriate sentence for this crime you say you've committed?

Is it a life sentence? Would you place this sentence on anyone else who has shared your experience? I doubt it.

Still others equate acceptance with forgiveness and feel that they just can't do that, because forgiving others is equated to making it OK. Accepting what happened to you does not make it OK. Not at all. Acceptance does not mean that what happened was right and fair and just. Some things that happen to us can never be OK and will always be absolutely terrible and unfair. Acceptance means that you understand it, you recognise it, you see it, you name it, and you are able to move on rather than dwell on it or deny it.

It's all very well me saying that reaching acceptance on the other side is peaceful, but if you've never experienced it, I understand that it feels like a risk. What I can tell you is that everyone I've ever spoken to has said it's worth it.

Asking you what you're in denial about may seem like a strange question, after all, surely if you're in denial you don't know you're in denial! But oftentimes you do know, deep down, and that's the feeling I'm asking you to connect with here. What are you in denial about? What losses have you not yet grieved? What experiences have you shut off? What emotions do you pretend you don't feel? What comes up for you when you read about acceptance? Anything you name that you have a strong reaction to is likely to be a sign that you're looking in the right place.

Projection

Projection is another defence mechanism that is becoming more common in general conversation. Projection occurs when we push our own unwanted thoughts, feelings and motives onto somebody else thereby transferring the ownership of these feelings to another person. One example would be a cheating husband who suspects his partner is being unfaithful. By projecting we can avoid having to consciously identify, take ownership of, and deal with our thoughts and emotions. We shift the blame, and our focus is on someone else instead of ourselves. The cheating husband knows that he is in the wrong, but rather than face his actions he accuses his wife of doing the same. If we are insecure about our bodies, we might spend more time judging others and making comments around other people's bodies to distract attention away from ourselves.

Assumptions

We all have a tendency to make assumptions about other people. In particular, we tend to assume that other people think, feel and react the same way that we do. Spoiler alert: they don't. In clinic, this can present as a problem when people assume that others around them will judge and shame them for their eating, or their body, because they do it to themselves. We don't trust others because we don't trust ourselves. Yes, our past experiences can and do play a role, but so do our projections of the way we feel about ourselves on to others.

Rationalisation

Rationalisation is a popular defence mechanism among those I see who are particularly intelligent. Some see rationalisation as an excuse; I see it as more of a deflection of emotions. It is used by people to avoid having to focus on feelings and to instead rely on logic. Again, this is not done consciously and deliberately, but as an automatic process the brain employs to protect you from the potential pain and overwhelm of your emotions. Logically, we can know one thing, but internally in our core we can believe something entirely different. I spend a fair amount of time with very logical and rational clients asking them to temporarily set aside their rational brain. I say to them, 'OK, now we've heard from the rational you, can that part take a step back please and then can the emotional you step forward and answer as well?' Someone who has been sexually assaulted can logically know it's not their fault, but if deep down they believe that they have done something to deserve it, that will win over every single time. That is what will influence their thoughts and behaviours. But that belief is often a much more uncomfortable truth, so we rationalise to cover it up, which helps us seem like we make more sense to ourselves and others. This isn't helped by people around us who will say things like, 'How can you believe something like that?' Or, 'Surely you must know that's not true, right?' Logically yes. We know it. But emotionally, if we believe differently, that has greater power.

If you're struggling with this, imagine your logical brain and emotional core as two characters. What would they say to each other? Where would they differ in their outlook on your experiences? When you let them each have their space and their say, without your logical brain talking over your emotional core, you may be surprised at what you hear.

Like all defence mechanisms, rationalisation has its place and function in protecting us. But it gets in the way of us perceiving a better, healthier relationship with food and ourselves because it doesn't allow us to access our emotions and what we truly believe about ourselves. Until we are able to acknowledge our core beliefs, we cannot work through them. Until we acknowledge our emotions, no matter how uncomfortable they might be, we are not going to stop using food or any other mechanism as a method of suppressing our emotions.

Social comparison

Although Anna Freud did amazing work at defence mechanisms, one she didn't come up with was social comparison. As humans, we have a natural tendency to compare ourselves with others – it is a means of self-evaluation. This has great benefits in that it allows us to have an understanding of our social standing. In small doses, comparing ourselves to those who are slightly better than us can be motivating and drive our ambition. This is known as upward social comparison. In large doses, however, it can be harmful, demotivating and depressing. Similarly, in small doses, downward social comparisons help us to feel a little better about ourselves. A little comparison can help us to see ourselves more accurately, but a lot of comparison hurts almost everyone.

If we give too much weight to our comparisons to others and how they may perceive us as a result, our evaluation and main definition of success is coming from an external place. This is incredibly unstable in the long run, and so fragile, as it gives others great power over us. Too much upward social comparison can reinforce our belief that we're not good enough. If you have high self-esteem, upward social comparisons are unlikely to affect you that much. In fact, they're more likely to offer you hope and motivation. If, however, your self-esteem is already low, then a lot of upward social comparisons will only make you feel worse.

Both my clinical experience and several academic studies show that those who are perpetually on a diet are more likely to be influenced by comparison with what others are eating.[26] Dieters are more likely to be concerned about what others around them are eating, more likely to use them as a guide, and more likely to beat themselves up if they feel that their food behaviours are not up to scratch. Those with food freedom who have positive body image are actually far less likely to engage in that kind of comparison or to internalise a sense of their worth based on any comparison.

Those who are struggling with an eating disorder or disordered eating may find their recovery hindered by excessive comparison. Research shows that body image and food comparison in particular drives behaviours such as restriction and binge eating.[27] I would definitely not go so far as to say that comparison causes these behaviours, but it does seem to contribute to their maintenance rather than recovery.

I have seen what people are capable of when they spend less time comparing themselves to others. I have seen how they are able to grow, thrive and do wonderful things for themselves. When this barrier is removed, there is so much that people realise they're capable of, and their motivation is so much more powerful.

There is also a lot of power in selecting an appropriate comparison target. If someone has a close friend, family member or partner in their life who has a great relationship with food, they can be an amazing role model. I have encouraged people to engage in a little bit of comparison in this way, as this can help people motivate themselves to move closer to that healthier relationship with food.

Defence mechanisms are strong barriers, and they can be helpful or unhelpful, and the degree of their usefulness can change with time. They are strong walls that we put up to protect ourselves from others and from ourselves. They are the walls around our castles. The stronger they are, the more they protect us in times of need. But in times of peace, when the threat has passed, they remain there. Just in case. We feel as if we're still protecting ourselves, but really we're keeping other people out. For some of us, that includes keeping ourselves out too. It can even involve a disconnection between the brain and the body to the extent that you struggle to notice emotions, hunger or even the cold.

8

Alexithymia

Some of my clients who have experienced trauma, or who have been taught by significant figures in their life to suppress their emotions, or that their emotions are bad, find difficulty in recognising what it is they are feeling. In extreme cases, it's as if their brain and body are disconnected from one another. This is known as alexithymia, which is a difficulty or an inability to recognise or name emotions with words. It can also been described as emotional blindness.

Roger, who I mentioned in Chapter 2, faced significant abuse at the hands of his parents. Early on in our conversations, I noticed that he didn't really talk about how he felt. He was very narrative driven, a great storyteller, but it was like he was talking about someone else. Then one day he arrived late to one of our sessions. It had been raining and he had been walking in the rain with no gloves and no raincoat, yet he said he felt fine. He didn't notice that his hands were so frozen he could barely move them. I brought this up with him to try to understand what was going on for him, and it turns out that he was so disconnected from his body that he couldn't feel the cold at all. He returned the following week looking much more subdued and reflective. He said to me, 'If I separate myself from my body, I separate myself from the hurt that was caused to me.' This was his way of coping, his way of surviving. It's an extreme kind of out-of-body experience.

If you remember the various trauma responses we discussed earlier, we have fight, flight, freeze and fawn (page 40). Those who experience freeze (which occurs due to an inability to fight or run away) are more likely to experience a sense of disconnection from the body, because it feels unsafe to be present and alert in your body. This is a form of dissociation, and is often experienced by survivors of rape and sexual assault precisely because it disconnects you from your body as a way of coping.

Those who have not experienced trauma may still have great difficulty recognising, naming and processing our emotions, especially if we've had our emotions dismissed, ridiculed or invalidated at a young age. This is a significant barrier that can prevent us from being able to work towards a healthier relationship with food that is not so emotionally charged. If we have difficulty recognising our emotions, how can we meet our own needs? How can we give ourselves what we actually need in the times when we are seeking something else that isn't food?

Looking inward

Connecting with and recognising our emotions is an introspective experience. It requires looking inward within ourselves to find the answers to the question, 'what's going on right now?' If we have difficulty doing this with our emotions, we may also have a similar experience with other aspects of bodily awareness, whether that's our heart rate, tiredness, or even hunger and thirst signals. If you struggle to differentiate between emotional states – for example confusing anger and sadness – you might also have difficulty discerning hunger – for example confusing hunger and thirst,[28] or confusing emotional and physical hunger. Butterflies in the stomach due to anxiety might be mistaken for physical hunger, and vice versa.

When we have interoceptive awareness (the ability to identify, access, understand and respond appropriately to the patterns of internal signals), we can absolutely tell the difference between these because we have that connection with our body and the signals it's sending to our brain about what's going on and what we need.* This is useful information, as it enables us to take better care of ourselves, and it builds trust with our body. In research, alexithymic individuals tend to have less energy, poorer emotional well-being, poorer social functioning, more pain and poorer general health than those without alexithymia.[29] (I discuss interoceptive awareness further in Chapter 14.)

Pause for a moment right now, and notice what's going on in your body. Can you feel your heart beating without placing a finger on your pulse? Can you tell if you're hungry, full, or neither? Where does your body feel tired or sore? What emotions are you experiencing right now, and where in your body do they live? Give yourself a minute or two to try to answer. If you struggle, you're probably someone who could benefit from greater interoceptive awareness.†

Alexithymia and eating disorders

It's probably not surprising that alexithymia is more common in individuals with eating disorders than in the general

---

* It's important to note that there is a relationship between autism and alexithymia, so if you're not neurotypical, that may also be playing a role here.
† Alexithymia is not yet a formal diagnosis, and I'm not here to diagnose you when I haven't met you!

population.[30] In other words, those with eating disorders have greater difficulty with identifying and describing their emotions compared to your average person without an eating disorder. Also, the more eating-disorder behaviours someone engages with and the more often those occur, the more likely they are to have higher levels of alexithymia. Behaviours like bingeing, purging, restriction and over-exercising are all ways to either avoid or cope with emotions. On top of that, there can then be secondary emotions such as shame, guilt or disgust around experiencing an emotion or around the behaviour itself; for example, you may feel angry, so you overeat and purge, and then feel shame and disgust at having overeaten and purged. Or you may feel jealous and then feel guilty for feeling jealous. Or shame at feeling anger, or any other combination you can think of. More behaviours usually equate to greater difficulty with emotions.

This fits with both what the research shows and what my own clinical experience suggests: those with anorexia have higher alexithymia levels and difficulty expressing emotions, which may be due to the numbness that is often experienced in a restrictive and semi-starvation state, alongside the high that individuals can experience when facing intense hunger. Those with bulimia, emotional eating and overeating still have high alexithymia levels, but not the same degree as those with anorexia. This likely has something to do with the secondary emotions like shame, guilt and disgust, which, due to our societal conditioning around eating and weight gain, may be more likely to appear after overeating. What both avoiding eating and overeating in response to emotions have in common is often a sense of overwhelm, of unidentified emotions running high, and using food to cope. Words such as 'overwhelmed', 'bad' or 'weird' are often cover words for the emotions someone is experiencing, which may be either too uncomfortable or too elusive to name. When someone says 'I feel weird', they may truly mean 'I feel anxious'. Saying 'I feel bad' can mean 'I feel upset and frustrated.' If someone is overwhelmed, I wonder: overwhelmed by what? Is there too much anger? Sadness? Fear? A combination of several? Finding out helps us to move forward with finding specific coping mechanisms for that feeling.

Carla developed alexithymia due to a trauma in early adolescence, which taught her that her body wasn't her own, and she shut down her emotional experiences. She would regularly say to me, 'I feel like a robot', meaning that she was going through the motions, getting her work done (she was a perfectionist too), and not really recognising her emotions. When we first met, she would speak with a relatively flat, inexpressive voice and would never cry, even when discussing difficult topics. I'm generally able to tell quite easily if someone is about to cry or is trying to hold back tears, but I got nothing from her for many months. She was a great storyteller and wonderfully introspective when it came to her thoughts and beliefs, but emotions were much more of a challenge, particularly shame. Part of her recovery from her disordered eating involved becoming, in her words, less of a robot and more of a human.

The role of shame

Shame and alexithymia have an especially interconnected relationship due to how powerful a feeling shame is, how all-encompassing it is, and how it can eat away at us for so many years. In Carla's case, the shame around what she had experienced as a teenager was a significant contributor to her disconnection from emotions. When researchers mapped where we feel emotions in our body, shame is the one that people primarily noticed in their head, a little in the chest, and a numbness in the rest of the body. In this way, feeling shame encourages a disconnect between brain and body through the physical sensations it evokes.

Alexithymia isn't simply something that occurs coincidentally alongside an eating disorder. Sometimes it is a contributing factor to the development of eating issues beyond diagnosable eating disorders. If someone has experienced physical and emotional abuse or neglect in childhood, the messages around their self-worth and their emotions may lead to alexithymia and a difficulty expressing emotions, which may then lead to food as a means of coping. When we have been taught not to feel certain emotions, when we can't find the words to express what we feel, it's not surprising that we channel that into something physical like food.

Emotions live in our body, memories are stored in our body, and food becomes our body. It's no wonder that they are all connected. We attach a huge number of assumptions and judgements of morality and worth to our bodies, and so when we experience emotions that are unacceptable to us, we associate that with our body where that emotion lives, and we disconnect. Feeling like you don't understand and can't describe what's going on in your body only exacerbates this further, increasing the likelihood of feeling frustrated with your body for not making sense to you. This is not conducive to positive body image, instead leading to a reinforcing of the body as the problem.

Name your emotions

When clients come to me saying they want help with emotional eating, I often ask them to tell me which emotions they use food to cope with. Many are unable to answer, or instead they tell me about situations and events rather than feelings. I've had clients sitting in front of me crying, and when I ask them what's going on for them, they don't know. When you don't like something or don't understand it, you distance yourself from it, and we do the exact same with our bodies. The greater your difficulty with emotions, the more likely you are to also dislike your body. What this also means is that working on recognising and naming your emotions can improve your body image.

There is also a relationship between alexithymia and perfectionism, both of which can increase the risk of an eating disorder, and which we'll be discussing next.

If you struggle to describe and express your emotions, this likely presents a barrier that is preventing you from reaching the relationship with food you want. Like with all barriers, dismantling it leads to progress. We can do this by increasing our awareness of our emotions, finding ways to communicate and verbalise how we feel, and by understanding what our emotions are telling us.

9

Perfectionism

Perfectionism is misunderstood. It's seen as a humble brag – a strength disguised as a weakness. A lot of people say to me, 'I can't be a perfectionist, I don't do anything perfectly', but that's actually not how perfectionism works. There is a positive side to perfectionism, in that it can allow us to be ambitious, aim high and achieve great things in life. It can be an incredible driver towards success. Above all, there is pleasure at working hard at something, and pride in one's achievements, but there is also flexibility. This form of perfectionism is known as 'adaptive perfectionism'. It's healthy, it's useful and it's productive. Maladaptive perfectionism, however, is a little different. The thought patterns behind maladaptive perfectionism are typically all-or-nothing self-critical thinking ('If I eat one bad thing I've failed'), repeatedly using 'should' and 'must' ('I should be able to avoid chocolate all the time'), and fear of failure ('If I don't do well others will think I'm useless').

All-or-nothing thinking is also often called black-and-white thinking, due to a notable absence of middle ground or grey. You might identify with this if you're the kind of person who says, 'Fuck it!' and eats an entire box of cookies after you've had two because you might as well eat the whole lot now so that they're gone, and besides your 'plan' or 'goal' or 'diet' is ruined anyway so why not eat the whole box? Fuck it!

Our fear of failure

Underlying the above thoughts are assumptions and beliefs about ourselves; for example, 'If I don't eat perfectly, then I'll become unwell', or 'If I eat more, then I am greedy', or 'If I don't succeed, then I'm a worthless person.' These assumptions tend to be rigid and inaccurate, making them particularly damaging to our self-esteem.

Sometimes it shows up in clinic in the form of people trying to achieve the perfect diet. Sometimes it shows up in very rigid, all-or-nothing thinking, such as 'If I am thin, my life will be perfect and everything will fall into place', in beliefs such as 'If I don't do well, others will think I'm lazy and useless', or 'If I don't get everything right in my job, I'll get fired'. There is a great deal of fear that drives these beliefs and behaviours, which creates a great barrier to change. Fear is powerful. Notice how in all these beliefs people are running away from something: failure. Despite perfectionism being the pursuit of success, it's really more defined by a fear of failure. They're running away from failure rather than running towards achieving something, because what perfectionists are running towards – namely total perfection – doesn't actually exist.

Perfectionism can show up in your thoughts and words in a number of ways; for example:

- 'I strive to be the best at everything I do.'
- 'I can't leave something until I've triple-checked it for any mistakes.'
- 'Others won't like me if I don't succeed.'

- 'People around me expect me to be good at everything.'
- 'I have to do well, otherwise I'm a failure.'
- 'If someone brings up a mistake I've made, I feel embarrassed, ashamed and like I've failed.'

This last one is generally a good litmus test for perfectionism in my experience. Imagine you've made a mistake and someone has pointed it out to you. How do you respond? Do you say 'Oops!' and thank them for catching it? Do you blush and feel a bit embarrassed but get over it? Or does it linger in your mind for weeks or even months, leaving you feeling like you're an idiot, and now everyone around you thinks you're an idiot, so you're never going to get that promotion, and my God, why can't you do a single thing right, now you have to make sure you work even harder to get it just right next time. If you react in the latter way, you may just be a perfectionist, or at the very least you have a maladaptive perfectionistic thinking style. If your self-worth is tied to your ability to achieve in this way, it places you in a particularly vulnerable position, where your worth can easily be shattered by a single mistake.

This maladaptive perfectionism has a number of downsides that you might experience. See if you identify with any of the following:

- I have no free time.
- I don't take time to celebrate achievements because I could always do better, and there's always more to do.
- I blame myself if things aren't done just right.
- I must do everything right the first time.
- I have to go over my work many times until it's acceptable to my standards.
- I struggle to make decisions in case it's the wrong choice.

- I'm so afraid of failing that I procrastinate and struggle to get started.
- I give up on something if I can't do it well right from the start or if I made a mistake.

Unhelpful rules for living

Perfectionism leaves us with these damaging effects, thanks to assumptions and rules for living that drive our behaviour. A rule or assumption tends to be unhelpful when it is inaccurate and inflexible in some way; for example, Hazel (who we met in Chapter 2) became a perfectionist partly due to never getting praise or approval from her father. In adulthood, she worked long hours, often being the first to arrive at work and the last to leave, and she missed out on spending time with her children. If anything went wrong in the company, she would blame herself; if something needed to be done, she'd do it herself rather than delegate; and if someone asked her for help, she would always say yes. Her initial accurate belief of 'people like it when I help them' became an inflexible rule of 'I must help people otherwise they won't like me', and led her to consistently help others at the expense of her own free time and well-being. Once we identified what her rules and assumptions were (hint: they usually begin with 'I should ...' or 'I must ...') we were able to work through them and gradually shape them into something less rigid.

Diane was also someone who worked long hours as part of her perfectionism, and it showed up very clearly in her relationship with food in the form of all-or-nothing thinking. She would have a couple of days where she was very rigid and planned with food, then she would have one meal out or a few glasses of wine and switch into 'fuck it!' mentality. What would follow was a few days of racking up a significant bill on food delivery apps and eating until she felt painfully full. Whenever this happened her inflexible beliefs showed up – 'I should be able to stop this', 'I'm a failure' – and tormented her until she felt awful about herself. Her maladaptive perfectionism would lead her to give up on herself when she couldn't immediately get everything right. I lost count of how many times Diane claimed that she had given up on our work together only to show up again a few weeks later.

The rise of perfectionism

I work with people of all ages between sixteen and eighty. Perfectionism can manifest at any age, but I particularly see huge numbers of young people – Millennials and Gen Zs – struggling with perfectionistic beliefs. This isn't surprising when you consider that the American Psychological Association has found that perfectionism among young people has increased significantly since the 1980s.[31] This rising perfectionism is likely contributing to an increase in anxiety and depression among younger generations, due to their exhausting and relentless inner critic putting them down, and their persistent anxiety and fear around failure.

There is also a link between perfectionism and eating disorders. There is the clear connection, as seeking total perfection includes seeking the 'perfect' body, which is achieved through the food that's eaten, as well as a sense of being in total control of your life. Eating-disorder pioneer and psychoanalyst Hilde Bruch described young patients with anorexia nervosa as fulfilling 'every parent's and teacher's idea of perfection', as they often aim for perfect grades and being a perfectly compliant child who always does their homework and chores without any confrontation. To some, this might appear like they're the 'ideal' child or student. Children and adolescents who display strong tendencies of perfectionism are far more likely to develop disordered eating. Most people with anorexia score highly on perfectionism, both in terms of high standards towards the self as well as believing that others expect perfection from them. Perfectionism acts together with low self-esteem and poor body image to raise someone's risk of an eating disorder, and it also seems to make recovery more challenging. Individuals who have recovered from an eating disorder will often still have higher levels of perfectionism than the average person without an eating disorder, even sixteen years after the initial diagnosis.[32] This could be because in recovery there is often more a focus on weight restoration rather than reducing psychological symptoms, and because perfectionism is so ingrained and even encouraged, not just with food but also in many areas of life. It is rare for someone to have perfectionistic tendencies when it comes to food and nothing else.

Every perfectionist I meet, whether they have a diagnosed eating disorder or not, has a strong inner critic that tells them they're never good enough. We will cover this more in the next chapter, but for now I'd like you to consider this: we often think that self-criticism is helping us because it drives us. But the very notion of adaptive perfectionism – a flexible rather than all-or-nothing way of thinking – suggests that that's not necessarily the case. As the classic analogy goes, if you want a donkey to carry your stuff up a hill, you can either hit it with a stick or you can encourage it with a carrot. Either way, that donkey is going up the hill, but when there's a stick involved that donkey is going to be much more miserable than when there's a carrot. As a recovering perfectionist myself, I struggled for a long time with the idea that I don't have to beat myself up in order to get things done. I resisted that idea for so long because I was so entrenched in my way of thinking, which to be fair, had taken me pretty far in life. But at what cost? I took a leap of faith and tried using more of a reward-based system – like a carrot. Strangely enough, I'm just as productive as ever, and I'm happier too. Perhaps it's time to trust that you can do the same.

Perfectionism and emotional eating

It's clear that perfectionism is a barrier that prevents people from pursuing a better relationship with food. In fact, research shows that negative or maladaptive perfectionism increases the likelihood that someone will be an emotional eater.[33] Perfectionism comes with a lot of stress and difficult thoughts and emotions, which are challenging and can be avoided or suppressed with food.

Food is not simple and straightforward, food is not good or bad, and one food or meal doesn't have the power to make you a good or bad person, but we continue to speak as if it does. This idea that one food can undo your entire pursuit of health is unhelpful and untrue. Moreover, the more we tell ourselves that we can't have a food because it is bad, the more our brains want it because it brings that food right to the forefront of our minds. Nutrition is complex and context dependent, but black-and-white thinking does not allow us to really appreciate that or understand food in this way. Instead, we boil it down into some oversimplification that doesn't do food justice. It gets in the way of enjoying, appreciating and celebrating food.

As you try to improve your relationship with food, those perfectionistic thoughts will get in your way, especially when (not if) you make some kind of mistake or slip up, or things don't quite go your way. They inevitably will, because any kind of recovery is never linear. A maladaptive perfectionist at this point is more likely to say, 'What's the point? It doesn't work,

I failed. I'm a terrible person. I can't do this' and abandon the idea. Or potentially, a mistake is made, you feel embarrassed and upset, you feel like you're a failure, and this makes it so much harder to continue the process because it becomes a self-fulfilling prophecy. If you're not speaking to yourself kindly, it becomes considerably more challenging to act kindly towards yourself because all your thoughts and beliefs are telling you that you don't deserve it, not just when it comes to food but in every aspect of your life. This is why tackling and reshaping perfectionistic thoughts and beliefs is such an integral part of recovery from any kind of eating concerns and can help bring more contentment to your life as a whole.

If you identify with the statements or stories I've shared here, I encourage you to just sit with them a little. We will come to strategies and tools to help reshape your maladaptive perfectionism into a more adaptive form later. It's important that we stay with what we observe and identify for a moment before rushing to solutions. Particularly as perfectionism often appears together with another significant barrier to a healthy relationship with food and yourself: a strong self-critical voice.

10

Self-Critical Voice

Do you have that little voice in your head that tells you you're not good enough? If so, you're not alone in that. Many of us have an internal monologue comprised of several voices that can talk to each other. One of those voices might be a self-critical voice. In some people it's the loudest voice they have.

During my initial conversation with a new client, I can usually spot quite quickly those people who have a very loud self-critical voice. They're very hard on themselves ('I'm just lazy'), self-blaming ('I don't have enough self-control') and use the word 'should' a lot ('I should be able to stop doing this'). They beat themselves up for not being where they want to be in life. Often, they beat themselves up for overeating or eating for emotional reasons. They talk to themselves in a way that they would never dream of talking to anybody else in their life. Yet, because this process is internal, they often don't even question the fact that they are being so cruel to themselves.

When I notice this, I usually make a point of mentioning it pretty quickly. 'I've noticed you are really hard on yourself', I tell them. This usually produces one of two responses, either 'I hadn't noticed' or 'I know, but it's necessary.' Either they are unaware of it, or they feel it's justified.

I hear a lot of people tell me that they should just be able to stop stress eating or emotional eating or restricting or binge-ing. I understand where they're coming from, but clearly they are struggling. If they could do it alone, they would have done it by now. If it were as simple as expecting it to stop, then they wouldn't be talking to me. 'Should' is just 'could' with judgement attached, after all. 'Could' suggests options, possibility, an empowered choice, an internal drive and desire. 'Should' comes from a place of obligation, an external judge and authority telling you what to do. I see 'could' as a hand outstretched in invitation, whereas 'should' is a derogatory wagging finger. The people I meet aren't lazy or lacking willpower; they have significant barriers in the way that prevent them from pursuing what they want for themselves. That's why we work on dismantling them.

I usually start this process by inviting someone to be curious about what their self-critical voice is doing for them. We discuss what they might be afraid will happen if their self-critical voice went away or wasn't so loud. I'm not looking for a logical answer, but an emotional answer that comes from the voice itself. Usually, what comes up is that the self-critical voice is actually trying to protect them, and they worry that if it wasn't so loud, they would end up doing something that made them look bad, or they wouldn't try hard enough and would fail. Often, when this voice is loud and yells it's because the voice learned this behaviour from parents, caregivers or other authority figures. If these figures in life were loud, critical and, at the same time, seemingly successful in helping the person achieve, the self-critical voice adopts those mannerisms with the assumption that this drive and success will continue. By discussing this we can reach a point where instead of thinking that the voice criticising them is out to get them, they realise that the intention is to protect, while understanding both where that voice originated and who it is echoing. That doesn't mean that it has to stick around exactly as is, simply that they understand, which means that we can work with it.

A critical defence

The self-critical voice usually appears alongside defence mechanisms. If we have a parent who is unable to meet our needs on a regular basis, either physically or emotionally, we may develop a sense of 'I don't need anyone else', and alongside that the self-critical voice emerges and says 'you're too needy' as a way of interpreting this rejection. The voice supports the defences to create a coherent narrative. A reminder that as children we tend to believe that what happens to us is our fault because we are dependent on our parents to nurture us, and we need to believe that our parents can take care of us. The parent has to be good and able, which makes us bad or at fault. And so a self-critical narrative is born, which tells you that you're not good enough out of self-protection, because the idea that our parents can't take care of us is too devastating to comprehend while we're children.

The self-critical voice is a barrier that's preventing you from letting go of old thinking patterns that no longer serve you. After pointing it out to clients, I often ask them, 'What do you gain from being so hard on yourself?' Or 'What do you gain from having such a strong self-critical voice?' The common responses I get are around it being motivating, or the idea of, 'If I'm harder on myself then I'll stop stress eating.' It's a punishment-based system, because somewhere along the line they've been taught that this is the best way to get something done.

Sure, being self-critical can be motivating, but that doesn't mean it's the only way. Remember that donkey from the last chapter that we're trying to get up the hill? You can beat it with a stick (self-criticism) or you can dangle a carrot in front (self-kindness). The stick, your self-critical voice, gets you up the hill – but at what cost?

The idea of being hard on yourself as a deterrent is flawed logic. If it really were an effective deterrent, you wouldn't keep repeating the cycle of overeating (or avoiding eating if you tend towards restriction), beating yourself up for it and overeating again soon after. But you do. It's not serving you in the way that you want it to. It's not actually an effective method of prevention, so maybe it's time to let it go. Perhaps it's time to at least give it less power and to try something else. Being kind to yourself can be just as motivating, so why not give yourself a carrot? The way I see it, you have nothing to lose. The worst that could happen is nothing changes. The best that could happen is that you're genuinely kinder to yourself and therefore happier.

Perfectionistic critics

The self-critical voice is heavily tied to perfectionism, so if you're a perfectionist, you likely have a strong self-critical voice too. When you are trying desperately to do everything perfectly, the self-critical voice tells you that you're not good enough, because you've fallen short of an impossible goal. Perfectionists rarely feel good enough. One of the hallmarks of perfectionism is never being satisfied with achievements or even the effort put into them, due to unrealistic expectations. Then, when you inevitably fail to meet those expectations, it serves as further evidence that you're not good enough. Perfectionists meet this sense of failure with harsh self-criticism.

You might think that being hard on yourself is necessary, as if it will motivate you to do better. But criticism usually leads to shame, not to greater motivation. In other words, criticism makes us feel worse about ourselves, and we can't grow and do better when we're too busy putting ourselves down.

I had a strong self-critical voice for most of my life, which was intertwined with my perfectionism. I thought that it was an incredibly important part of my motivation, my drive, my ambition, and my success. I thought that if I let it go, I would begin to slide backwards. I had been relying on my self-criticism to keep me in check for so long that I couldn't imagine getting anywhere without it. The fear of losing my drive to succeed kept me exactly where I was: hard on myself, never celebrating my successes, always moving straight on to the next thing. It took my therapist regularly poking at this idea for months for it even to begin to shift. I can see the change simply in how I'm writing this book. Rather than pushing myself to keep writing and keep writing, I set myself a target for the day – my carrot dangling in front of me. And when I reach that target, no matter what time of day it is, I take that carrot, I acknowledge my achievement, and I relax. Sometimes that means I'm writing for eight hours. Sometimes it means I'm writing for three. My drive has not gone, it is just as alive as ever, and I am more content than before.

If you have an active inner monologue, a literal voice in your head that talks to you throughout the day, it gives you a wonderful opportunity to notice the way you speak to yourself as an observer and to begin to interrogate whether there might be a kinder approach that you can take. Ask yourself:

- What does the voice say?
- In what tone (if it has one)?
- Does it say 'I' or 'you' or 'we'?
- Who does it sound like?

This last question often produces fascinating discussions in my clinical practice. I have met people who tell me that their inner self-critical voice sounds like their own, like their parents, or like a younger version of themselves. This often gives some insight as to where this voice has emerged from and what work may need to be done. In most instances, the self-critical voice will sound like you – after all, it's internal and part of the self. If you hear the voice of a parent, what was your relationship like? Do you have some unprocessed experiences in this relationship that you would benefit from working through? If you hear the voice of a younger version of you, perhaps you as a child, it might mean that your inner child still has some unmet needs. What do they need? Can you find a way to give yourself that now as an adult?

Inner experiences

Of course, not everyone has an internal monologue, and even those who primarily do may still have thoughts that aren't verbal. In his years of studying the inner workings of people's minds, psychologist Russell Hurlburt has come up with five categories of inner experiences: inner speaking, inner seeing (real or imaginary), emotions, sensory awareness (such as feeling the carpet under your feet) and unsymbolised thinking. This last one can be a tricky concept to get your head around, but it is essentially a thought that doesn't manifest as words or images but is undoubtedly present in the mind.

Three of these inner experiences are clearly about thoughts: inner speaking (the inner monologue), inner seeing (visual focus) and unsymbolised thinking. While most of us will engage in all three, we tend to have a dominant form. If you have an inner monologue, prepare to have your mind blown: *some people don't experience this at all*. I would know, I'm one of them. My own mind was blown when I learned that the concept of the inner monologue wasn't just a literary plot device but actually a real thing that people experience.

If you have a very visual brain, you may find yourself experiencing an image or memory of a parent criticising you, or visualising people's disappointment in you. My visual clients have described picturing themselves having a conversation with a boss telling them that they made a mistake and themselves replying, 'I know I made a mistake, I'm an idiot', or visualising themselves looking in the mirror at their body and feeling disgusted at it, or picturing themselves failing at something in the future rather than hearing the words 'you're going to fail at this'. For others, it can be an image of themselves as small, awkward and embarrassed, rather than specific scenarios. Still others describe a combination of visuals and a voice shouting at them, while some of my most incredibly visual clients who would have strong images in any other scenario find themselves without any visual at all when it comes to self-criticism. One client told me, 'It's weird; in any other situation my thoughts would be images, but when my self-critical voice is loud, it's just a voice shouting at me that's impossible to ignore.'

If your predominant experience is unsymbolised thinking, you may still have a faint self-critical voice, or a loud one, or no voice at all. You may find that you need to do some translation work – that has been my experience of quieting my inner critic. Because it's a thought that is absolutely present but is neither visual nor verbal, I find translating it into words is the most helpful method of understanding it and working with it, either in therapy or in your own process. It allows you to say it out loud to experience how it feels to hear it, or to write it down and look at it externally from yourself. In fact, I recommend that everyone with a strong self-critical voice write their thoughts out, no matter their thinking style. Often, we are so used to this voice that we don't pay attention to the exact wording used, and there is something powerful and eye opening about seeing these thoughts outside of our own minds. Sometimes externalising them in this way helps us to see just how intense and cruel our self-critical voice can be. It also gives us an opportunity to consciously and deliberately add a kinder narrative. When your self-critical 'voice' isn't a voice at all but just a presence, it can be hard to notice it in the moment and see it for what it is. You may have to work a little harder to dismantle it than someone with a strong inner monologue.

No matter how your brain works, if you have a strong self-critical experience, it will hold you back and prevent your growth. That criticism tells you that you're not good enough, that you're too much, that you're a failure, that you're wrong. Hearing these things doesn't exactly motivate you to grow into a person who has a good relationship with food and themselves. We know that shaming and criticising doesn't inspire people to make healthier choices for themselves – it does the opposite. Shame and critique drive emotional eating and destructive behaviours, and they may lead you to isolate yourself rather than to seek help and support.

11

Boundaries

Boundaries are essential in life, but they aren't as well under-stood as they should be. If we've been taught to say yes to absolutely everything and always put other people's needs above our own, we never end up getting round to our own priorities and needs. Being a people-pleaser or having a lack of boundaries can make it so much harder to build a relationship with food that is positive and healthy. This is often one of the hardest con-versations I have to have with people in clinic, simply because a lot of us are afraid that setting a boundary with someone would be a confrontational and difficult conversation, and we are afraid of the consequences of doing so.

We may have learned this in life through being manipulated by others in our early relationships or through being taught that our needs aren't as important. Sometimes it's as simple as being taught that a woman's role is defined by her relationship to other people: mother, sister, wife. There is a strong gender divide pres-ent in people-pleasing such that women are much more likely to be people-pleasers due to society placing very different external expectations on men and women. A man who chooses a career over family is ambitious, whereas a woman who does the same is seen as selfish. We encourage our young boys to be assertive, while encouraging young girls to be 'nice'. Once you begin to notice these differences, you'll start to see them everywhere. But it's starting to shift, and boundaries are one reason why.

A people-pleaser is someone who generally puts themselves last and focuses a lot of time and attention on making others happy. They will sacrifice their own needs in favour of others. If you find yourself always agreeing with others rather than stating your own opinions, if you apologise for things that aren't your fault, if you really struggle with saying no, if you have a strong fear of rejection, you are probably a people-pleaser. Some people-pleasers go to such great lengths to look after others that they end up unwell and burnt out with no time for themselves. People-pleasers often have weak boundaries, or none at all.

Boundaries are personal

Boundaries are essential in defining what we find acceptable and what we don't. Michelle Elman, an accredited life coach and the queen of boundaries, defines boundaries as 'the way we teach others to treat us. They are how we communicate what is acceptable and what is not. They define where you end and another person begins. We need boundaries in order to protect ourselves from manipulation, gaslighting [manipulating someone psychologically into doubting their own sanity], disrespect, and abuse.'* There are many different ways we might set boundaries with someone, whether that's around how someone speaks to us or topics of conversation, or the time spent with them, or how they treat our possessions. Boundaries are inherently personal. What might be an important boundary

---

* I highly recommend her book, *The Joy of Being Selfish: Why you need boundaries and how to set them.*

for me to set might be completely irrelevant to your situation. That's the thing about boundaries. Nobody can really tell you whether your boundaries are right or wrong, or whether they are too strict or too lenient. They are about protecting yourself and learning to put yourself first every once in a while, because there's nothing wrong in being a little bit selfish.

A lot of us have a difficult relationship with the word 'selfish'. We see it as an inherently bad thing, whereas being selfless is a good thing that is praised and encouraged. Selfless deeds are wonderful, but a lot of people who are seen as selfless are actually simply afraid to ask for what they need. They're afraid of the repercussions of it. It's about being liked by others.

Often this comes from childhood. In Chapter 2 we met Hazel. Her father was an alcoholic, and whenever she heard the sound of the key in the door, she didn't know which version of her father was coming home. It could be the angry drunk father or the kind but indifferent father. She learned to become so attuned to his mood and his needs through those early experiences that this fundamentally taught her to put others' needs above her own in order to protect herself. This kept her alive, but it now means that in adulthood she has few boundaries and lets people walk all over her. She is a classic example of someone who needed to learn to be more selfish. Her selflessness came from fear and self-preservation. Her needs were bottom of the priority list, but no one else was putting her first. The only person who was ever going to put her first was herself.

When our boundaries meet others

As my work with people focuses on their relationship with food and their bodies, the subject of boundaries is often introduced when people share how much people's comments around their body or what they're eating affects them. When we have endured years of others commenting on our bodies, asking people not to do so is often met with surprise or defensiveness. Whenever I have a conversation with someone in clinic about boundaries, I take great care not to sugar coat it: boundaries are hard. We can never predict how somebody else is going to respond to our boundary – there is no real way of knowing if they'll react well or badly. They may accept it and move on, or they may get defensive and angry and take it as a personal attack. How other people respond to you is outside of your control. What you can control is your intentions and your words. It's just like that dance-lesson scene in the movie *Dirty Dancing*: 'this is my dance space. This is your dance space.' My dance space is about me and my intentions; your dance space is about you and your reaction. They meet in the middle, but they are separate. Of course, this doesn't mean that our words have no meaning or no bearing on anybody else whatsoever. But even with the best intentions and the most carefully chosen words, we still cannot control exactly how someone responds to us setting a boundary, because how that person responds is a reflection on them and their life experiences, not you.

Let me give you an example. I have been told a few times in my life that someone finds me intimidating. Does this mean I objectively am intimidating? Not necessarily. I don't perceive myself as intimidating, it is not my intention to intimidate others, I'm just being me. At first when I was told this I assumed it was because I was too much. But then someone explained to me exactly why they found me intimidating. They said that I came across as intelligent and educated, which they found intimidating because they themselves did not attend university, even though they wish they could have. I was a physical representation of what they wish they had achieved. Clearly this had absolutely nothing to do with me and everything to do with that person's insecurities around their own education. I could have been anyone with a degree. It's not my fault if other people have insecurities that my mere presence elicits. Once that clicked, I stopped giving so much weight to whether people found me intimidating.

A lot of my clients who are parents find it easier to begin setting boundaries around their children than around themselves. For many people, it can be the stepping-stone they need to eventually be able to set boundaries with themselves. When it comes to their children, the concern is often around how comments about food and bodies might affect them. Often they themselves have experience of family members commenting on their bodies and on their food, and they've come to a place of awareness around how damaging this has been for them. Understandably, they don't want their kids to go through the same experience. The question then becomes, 'How do I ask my family not to comment on my children's weight or how much they are eating?' When I ask what's holding them back they usually say something about being concerned about hurting the other person's feelings.

It's common for my clients to have difficulties around boundaries with family that relate to food and their body. When Xena first set a boundary with her sister over the phone, they didn't speak for a few weeks. Her boundary was simple: 'Please stop asking me about my health every time we speak.' This was met with a great deal of defensiveness, ('I'm only looking out for you'), surprise ('Where is this coming from?'), and blame ('Well if you'd just lose weight, then I wouldn't have to keep worrying about you'). Xena stood firm the next time they spoke, when the usual health concerns came up, and maintained her boundary by saying, 'If you keep asking me about my health after I've asked you to stop, I will hang up.' And she did. She hung up every single time, and each time she would get an angry response from her sister via text with more blaming and defensiveness. It was a tough couple of weeks, but eventually her sister started respecting her boundary, and their relationship has been much better since.

Xena's sister clearly thought that this boundary was unreasonable, but that doesn't matter. Xena chose a boundary for herself, based on her experience and how she wanted to be treated, and it was an empowering moment for her. When you start setting boundaries, people around you may also tell you or imply that they don't agree with your boundaries, but it doesn't matter. Your life, your boundaries.

Of course, people can also respond well to our boundaries, and it's wonderful when that does happen. Caitlyn was a classic people-pleaser who took on other people's emotions and piled them on top of hers. When her husband was stressed out or feeling low, she would fixate on his feelings and try desperately to 'fix' them, as her anxiety was, 'If he's not OK then I'm not a good enough wife.' We discussed how this was part of a pattern she had developed of making other people's problems her own. She was able to recognise that this stemmed from a huge responsibility she felt as a child to take care of her father after her mother died. She expressed a desire to try taking a step back from making sure her husband was OK and set that boundary, and she quickly saw how they both benefited from this. After a few weeks of this she told me, 'My husband respects me so much more now, and I respect myself more too.'

Boundaries enable safety

I find the biggest misconceptions around boundaries is that they are fixed walls we put up to keep other people out. But there is a fundamental difference between a boundary and a wall.

Walls prevent any kind of closeness; they keep everyone out and they're usually built out of fear. Boundaries are designed to encourage vulnerability and closeness in a safe environment. They come from a place of self-love and self-respect, not fear.

When we engage in people-pleasing behaviour and have no boundaries, others may take advantage of us. At work, this might mean that people regularly ask you for help or delegate work to you because they know you won't say no. In relationships, it may mean that the other person knows they will always get what they want. In extreme cases it can also attract abusers. To be clear, I am not victim blaming. I do not blame the individual for being a people-pleaser or for not having boundaries. It is not their fault if they attract somebody abusive into their life. The blame always lies with the abuser. Nobody wants to attract somebody like that into their life on purpose. Nobody wants to have no boundaries. It's simply what we are taught. If that is our default position, any other seems unnatural and strange and as if it's too much.

Beginning to set boundaries with people who have been allowed to walk all over us is a risk. We risk losing those people, as they may not like how we've changed and grown. They may not like how we're finally putting ourselves first. It's a risk, but it is worth it. If someone no longer wants to be friends with you when they can no longer walk all over you, they are not your friend. You are better off without them in your life. If someone is friends with you only because they can take advantage of you, they're not a friend. They're using you, and you deserve better people in your life. Of course, all this is far easier said than done. The risk of losing people in our lives can be difficult to navigate and can prevent us from building a healthier relationship with food and ourselves. That risk and that fear holds us back and prevents us from pursuing what we want for ourselves. So many of us are afraid of being alone.

I often work with women whose friendships revolve around diet talk, or who work in offices where everyone is always on a diet. Once they stop dieting and try to establish a healthier relationship with food, they often find these same scenarios that they once enjoyed difficult to navigate. They often worry about being seen as boring or trying to be superior by not partaking in dieting. This is a good example of where people experience guilt after setting a boundary. That guilt is there because it is their brain saying they've done something wrong. But they haven't done anything wrong. The guilt is only there because they have been taught that they shouldn't be setting boundaries and shouldn't be putting themselves first, because they've been taught that this is a bad thing to do. In my experience, the more people set boundaries, the less guilt they experience afterwards. It does get easier.

Encountering resistance

An additional challenge in this environment is that those around you may be resistant to you changing. When those around us make the (in their eyes, very reasonable) assumption that you're in the same place you were before, it can feel like they're pulling you back to a past version of you. If someone is used to you constantly being on a diet, it may confuse them when you're no longer that person. Most of the time there's no malicious intent involved, just an awkward period of adjustment where your boundaries are needed, and you have to stand firm in yourself. That boundary shows those around you how you'd like to be treated from now on, and it is a sign of how much you value your relationship with someone.

Just because it's familiar and more comfortable to the people around you, it doesn't mean you have to undo your hard work and growth to accommodate them. They will adjust, or you'll compromise, or you'll part ways.

Improving your relationship with food means improving your relationship with yourself and that means learning to put yourself first. This requires you to learn more about what you actually *want*, rather than what you feel you *should* do and feel. If you're telling yourself that what you want doesn't matter enough, you're wrong. It matters a great deal, and it's time to start paying attention to that. Once you've figured that out, the next step is to be brave and communicate this to people.

In my experience, those who are unable to set boundaries end up in a cycle of repeating the same patterns over and over. They struggle to grow as a person, and the same concerns continue to come up in conversations, but nothing changes, because as long as you continue to passively put yourself last, nothing will change. It's only once you actively engage in putting yourself first and setting those boundaries that you'll see the change you're looking for in yourself.

Possible boundaries

These are the most popular boundaries my clients tell me that they want to set. Have a think about whether you may want them in your life too. You know you likely need to set these boundaries if you're finding that you wish you could talk about the following but feel uncomfortable at the idea of actually doing so:

- Boundaries around diet talk in front of the kids.
- Boundaries around discussing weight gain or weight loss.
- Boundaries around calling food good or bad.

- Boundaries around all body comments.
- Boundaries around commenting on portion sizes.
- Boundaries around the question 'should you be eating that?'

Of course, boundaries don't just have to be about not doing something. They can also be about adding something into your life, around stating your needs and how others can meet them; for example: 'I need you to include me in discussions around our weekly food shop', 'I need you to ask me if I'm hungry rather than just assuming', 'I need more physical touch and affection', 'I need you to talk to me when something is wrong', 'Sometimes I need you just to listen to me rather than offering me solutions.'

Always remember, boundaries are personal and individual. Although I've offered common ones that I see here, you have the power to decide which you'd like to set, and which ones you don't want or need. In Chapter 20 I suggest different practical ways in which you can set those boundaries.

12

Identity

'Who am I?' is a question we don't tend to ask ourselves very often.* It's a question that we instinctively feel we know the answer to yet struggle to express it when asked. I've not yet met someone who can quickly and articulately provide me with their answer when prompted.

Identity is an existential struggle. It is something we carry with us our entire lives and yet struggle to pin down with words. Do we have an inherent identity from birth that is unchanging and fixed? Is it something that we shape for ourselves throughout our lives? In reality, it is some combination of the two. Identity is something we inherit through birth (for example our race and culture), learn as we grow up, try on like clothes in adolescence, solidify in adulthood and shape with each experience that life throws at us.

I am fascinated by the existential concerns and dread that each human being faces at various points in our lives. My eyes light up whenever an existential question makes an appearance in the clinic room. We talk about having existential crises in terms of mid-life and quarter-life blips, laugh them off,

---

* Unless you're a big fan of *Les Misérables*, of course.

belittle them. But they are real and can teach us so much about ourselves.

The basic human existential concerns

Renowned psychotherapist Irvin Yalom describes four basic human existential concerns, or what many refer to as 'the ultimate concerns of human existence'. First is death and the inevitability of it. Second is freedom: the freedom to make our lives as we will, to be the sole author of our lives, thus leaving us being solely responsible. Third is existential isolation: we are born alone and die alone. Fourth is meaninglessness and the concern that we will have led a life without meaning.

I conceptualise these four concerns through four related questions I invite clients to answer:

- Death: what happens when we die?
- Freedom: what do I want?
- Isolation: who am I?
- Meaninglessness: what is my purpose in life?

To this I add a fifth question: Why me? – the question we ask ourselves when bad things happen, and we try to elucidate meaning from our experiences. Humans are unique in that we must learn to live and adapt to the realisation that we are mortal, our lives are finite.

Those who have experienced and overcome an identity crisis and those who feel they have found meaning in life tend to experience lower death anxiety due to a strong sense of self and accomplishment. Death anxiety is exactly what it says: an intense fear and anxiety about one's own death to the extent that it begins to interfere with everyday life. There is a very clear link between food and death. Food is what keeps us alive. If we don't eat enough or we don't eat at all, then we die. When the world around us feels uncertain and out of control, and the risks are so high as to include illness and death, some people turn to food as something to control that is certain. Among other reasons, fear of death drives people towards eating disorder behaviours and cognitions; however, paradoxically, death anxiety can also have positive effects. An awareness of our own mortality and fear of dying with regrets can drive us towards new learning and growth, acceptance, enhanced life meaning and the pursuit of an authentic existence.[34]

Realising that we will one day die can be a powerful driver that, when utilised for our benefit, can help us to figure out what we want (like a better relationship with food, for example) and who we want to be. Do you want to spend your finite existence stressing about everything you eat? Or is your time better spent with the joy and contentment of food freedom? Who are you and how does your relationship with food fit in with this?

Food and eating identities

When it comes to food and eating, the two identities or labels that I most often come across are 'the dieting one' and 'the healthy one'. What often tends to unite both of these is a concern about what other people will think. 'The dieting one' is the person who is always on a diet. Often they are in a larger body, and being the person who always diets serves several purposes as an identity. Firstly, it provides the narrative of the 'good fat person'. Being fat is seen as unacceptable in society, therefore the only way to make it somewhat OK is to be trying to move away from that state as much as possible and to be seen dieting and trying to make oneself smaller. Dieting helps us to avoid some sense of judgement from the people around us, because at least we are seen trying to lose weight and therefore obtain a socially acceptable body. It's a classic self-defence process. By taking on this identity and trying to make myself smaller, I protect myself from the judgement around me, because I'm already perceived to be judging myself for my size.

The second purpose this serves is a distraction from anything else going on in life. When dieting is your identity, it is immersive. Your headspace is taken up with thoughts of food and dieting. Your time is spent calorie counting and measuring out food. Your conversation is about the food you do and don't eat, how your diet is going, and how much weight you've lost. The process of dieting is so all-consuming that you don't need any other identity. In fact, you are actively discouraged from pursuing anything else. This also means that it's a beautiful distraction from any deeper existential concerns. As Michelle Allison, Canadian registered dietitian, so beautifully put it: 'This is why arguments about diet get so vicious, so quickly. You are not merely disputing facts, you are pitting your wild gamble to avoid death against someone else's.'[35] Diets are as personal as identity, and as powerful as religion.

We discussed the power of diets earlier in Chapter 3, Food and Love. I have met many people who, while they are dieting will not meet new people, find new hobbies or go on dates. They feel they must first lose weight before they can fully enjoy and embrace life. Often there is a fear that holds us back from trying new experiences, which goes beyond simply worrying what people think about our body – it can take us back to early childhood experiences. Not dieting means having to face the fears that are preventing someone from engaging in dating or other activities. The body is simply a more socially acceptable, convenient and physically obvious excuse. This doesn't take away from the fact that people in larger bodies are often judged when meeting new people. When engaging in any activities or when dating, that is very real and very present. In my clinical experience, however, there is also often something more deep-rooted at play, like a fear of rejection that stems from a parent leaving in early childhood. Focusing on weight and weight loss can be an excuse not to date, as the process of dieting is so all-consuming that it becomes a convenient distraction. Dating is seen as something that happens after the dieting is done, except that all too often the dieting is never done, because it's not about the end goal weight, it's about the process of dieting providing a distraction from the fear.

The identity of 'the healthy one' is often assigned to us by those around us. I have seen this more often in people in smaller bodies, although it can occur across the spectrum of weight and can overlap with 'the dieting one' identity. I see it most often in those who are struggling with orthorexia (the unhealthy obsession with eating what are considered 'healthy' foods). This doesn't have to be an identity you choose for yourself; as I pointed out above, sometimes it is given to you by those around you: 'Your lunches always look so healthy', 'You always pick the healthy option, don't you?', 'Look at you being healthy as usual.' When other people consistently assign an identity to us, we can easily adopt and internalise it and begin to develop a fear of not meeting their expectations.

Lara came to me due to concerns that her eating had tipped over from simply pursuing health to orthorexia. She had a history of disordered eating and struggled with her body image. She had taken on the identity of 'the healthy one' from a young age. When she was a teenager, Lara made the decision to be healthy by changing what she was eating and joining the gym. When she headed off to university, she joined Instagram and found a community of wellness bloggers and influencers, which reinforced her identity as 'the healthy one' and added greater restriction to her eating. When we first met, she said she didn't really identify with the diet culture cycle. In our first few months together, we discussed her various food fears and anxieties, and we planned to tackle them one by one. I sometimes ask people to complete a table or list of their food fears, as writing them down can help people clarify exactly what's going on. It puts it all in one place and allows people to add or take away items over time. It can be quite an experience for people to see all their food concerns listed on a page, and it can provide an incredible motivator for change.

When I asked Lara to talk through each of her food anxieties to try to understand where they had come from, she kept coming back to the pressure to be vegan. There was a real inner conflict in that she felt pressure to be doing as much as she could for the environment, while also recognising that due to her past disordered eating it was a risk. 'I know I shouldn't be vegan. It's not good for me. But at the same time I really feel like I should.' When she ate certain fear-foods such as dairy, it brought up thoughts around not being a good person and a feeling of disgust with herself. I knew at this point that it was time to dig deep into an exploration of health and identity. I could tell that this was a difficult topic for her, as it brought up tears very quickly. At first these tears were followed by frustration at herself; she didn't understand why this was producing such a strong reaction in her. But this was a deep-rooted identity that she had held on to for a long time, and she wasn't quite sure who she was without the focus on health. As with 'the dieting one' identity it was all-consuming and a distraction from her existential crisis. Our time together became focused on reshaping 'I don't know who I am without my food issues' into 'I am more than my diet.'

Teenage identities

Psychologist Erik Erikson's psychosocial stages of development state that adolescence is a time to explore identity, personal values, beliefs and goals. Adolescence involves a transition from childhood to adulthood and independence, and ideally in the process we are able to achieve an integrated sense of self and an idea of who we want to be in life. This is why you often see teenagers go through very intense phases such as fandoms and goth. I myself went through an epic boy-band phase as a teenager that lasted several years. It's worth reflecting back on this time in life and reminding yourself of how you threw yourself into one identity or another, like fashion or music or particular fandoms. How did these shape who you are today as an adult? Like many teenagers, you may have tried on several identities before you found one that stuck, and one of those identities may have been related to health. Unfortunately, this can become quite intense and obsessive to the point where it is all-encompassing and no other identities are tried. Lara is a clear example of this. She tried on 'the healthy one' identity as a teenager – it stuck around. Now she no longer knows who she is without it.

In the Pixar movie *Inside Out*, identity is portrayed beautifully in the form of islands, while the core emotions of joy, sadness, anger, disgust and fear live in the control centre of the protagonist Riley's brain. When they look out across the brain, they see Riley's islands of personality, like Family Island, Honesty Island and Hockey Island. Every time Riley loses one of these her identity begins to fade and she becomes depressed. If you haven't seen the movie, I encourage you to instead picture your identity as a pie chart. What do each of the slices represent? How many are there? How big is each one? Losing an eating disorder or the healthy identity or the dieting identity can feel like losing a large piece of the pie, leaving a gaping chasm. When you don't have very many slices to your pie, or when one is noticeably larger than all the rest, this can be a significant and painful loss. If your work is a key part of your identity you may feel depressed when you lose it. If exercise and moving your body define who you are, an injury could be devastating. This is why it is so important to add more to your sense of identity to soften the blow of a missing piece, whether that's friends, family, or interests and hobbies.

It's worth mentioning that identity and food are very closely linked. Even just the way we describe our patterns of eating is identity focused. We say 'I am vegan' or 'I am keto', not 'I eat vegan' or 'I eat keto.' It's not just something you do, it's something you are. For some, this may be absolutely true and a healthy part of a broad and varied identity. But it also makes it harder to let go when it no longer serves you. Letting go of an 'I am' is harder than letting go of an 'I do'. It's worth bearing this in mind when you talk about food and your relationship to it. Are you an emotional eater, or do you eat emotionally? Are you a chronic dieter, or have you simply been on many diets? How you define yourself is up to you, but it's something we don't often think about enough. I think it's worth choosing our words carefully when we are defining ourselves as a person. Especially if those words and that identity prevent us from growing into the person we want to be.

PART IV

TOOLS AND STRATEGIES FOR CHANGE

13

Solutions, Tools and Skills

Hopefully, through the preceding chapters you will have learned more about yourself, your relationship with food, and where any disordered eating and body image concerns might have come from. We've discussed a number of potential causes and contributors to difficult relationships with food and the body, as well as barriers that can prevent you from achieving the growth and change you're looking for.

If you're keen to engage in some deeper exploration on your own, I recommend reflecting and journaling around the following questions:

- What did I learn about my body as a child? How does this show up for me today?
- What did I learn about food as a child? How does this show up for me today?
- What did I learn about emotions as a child? How does this show up for me today?
- What did I learn about my worth and what I deserve as a child? How does this show up for me today?
- What did I learn about love as a child? How does this show up for me today?

The ultimate question here is: what are you really hungry for? What hunger is your emotional eating trying to solve with physical fullness? When you can answer that, once you learn to identify that hunger, to understand the conditions of worth that were placed on you, whether it's 'I am only loved if I am thin', or 'If I feel angry then I am bad and need to be punished', then you can start the process of unlearning those lessons and replace them with new ones. You can learn to recognise, sit with and express those emotions in constructive ways.

Please know that whatever your concerns are, they are valid, they are real, and you deserve to find a place of peace and happiness with yourself. Maybe you haven't experienced terrible trauma in life and wouldn't meet the criteria for a clinical eating disorder, but that doesn't mean you can't pursue some support and guidance. An ethical practitioner will never diminish or minimise your concerns, or compare them to other patients they see.

Therapy to reshape your brain

Alongside the above, you may want to consider whether exploring your past and your relationship with food in a formal environment is right for you. My favourite quick definition of what therapy is comes from chartered psychologist Kimberley Wilson, who writes, 'Therapy is a powerful, often challenging psychological intervention that can literally reshape the brain.' I think that's amazing – your brain isn't something fixed and unchanging; it's adaptable, constantly rewiring itself according to new experiences. No matter how old or young you are, you can change the shape of neural pathways and connections in your brain through the experiences you have in life, and what you choose to focus on. Every time you learn something new, or work towards unlearning something, your brain forms new connections, strengthens or weakens old ones, and adapts to the changes you make. This means that something as small as putting on clothes can become associated with focusing on what feels comfortable, rather than focusing on how your thighs look.

Therapy is about talking, yes, but it's also about building self-awareness, understanding your experiences in life and how they have shaped you today, and unlearning any unhelpful lessons you've been taught along the way. It is challenging, exhausting, frustrating, uncomfortable and so incredibly worthwhile. Sometimes therapy can feel like running an emotional marathon and hopefully an experience you'll be proud and grateful to have been through.

Whether or not you feel ready for therapy, I highly encourage engaging in your own self-reflection and self-exploration using the questions above, as well as anything that has come up for you in previous chapters. (See also the Postscript – Seeking Therapy or Nutrition Counselling.)

Tools to help you move forward

In the following chapters I will be offering you tools, skills and strategies to help you to dismantle your barriers and move towards a healthier relationship with food and your body. Every single one of the tools and skills I'm about to give you are ones I use with my clients in my clinical practice, and I have witnessed how impactful they can be. They are offerings, and it is up to you to try them, practise them, and take what works for you while casting aside what doesn't. If something feels uncomfortable, that is often a sign that you need it. If something feels unsafe, tread gently or take a step back. Some are simple, whereas others require dedicated time, patience and practice. After all, if you've been repeatedly putting yourself down, it's going to take more than a few days of being kinder to yourself for this to become a habit. It's like learning to drive a car: at first, every move you make is deliberate and conscious, but with practice and repetition it gradually becomes automatic, and you can drive while listening to music or having a conversation with someone. These tools are the same.

14

Interoceptive Awareness

When it comes to how we feel, we may have learnt in life that we can't trust our own experiences and our own bodies. We may have been taught to rely on external sources such as diet books ('eat these foods, but not these'), our parents ('you can't be hungry yet'), or the Internet ('maybe you're confusing hunger with thirst, so if you think you're hungry, have some water first!'). These messages, when repeated, and when told to us during moments of development or vulnerability, teach us that our bodies can't be trusted.

How to build trust

Diet culture capitalises on this lack of trust in ourselves, by selling us solutions that we can trust instead. Diets teach us that hunger is dangerous because you may overeat, that hunger can't be trusted because it might be thirst, and that hunger means you're out of control and you need to discipline your body into submission. Diet culture encourages us to suppress our hunger through drinking water or zero-calorie drinks, chewing gum or even smoking.

Our own life experiences may teach us that certain emotions are dangerous, undesirable, ugly, only acceptable when you're alone, or just plain wrong. These lessons teach us to suppress our emotions and avoid feeling them because they're unacceptable.

Do you see the problem?

Hunger is normal and human. Emotions are normal and human. There are no good or bad foods just like there are no good or bad emotions. Our bodies *can* be trusted. Yes, even yours.

We build trust with ourselves the same way we build trust with a stranger: with small moments of bravery and vulnerability. We wouldn't share our entire life story with someone we've just met (unless it's in therapy perhaps!), and we'd probably find it odd if someone was too open with us right from 'hello'. Equally, if someone is very closed-off and unwilling to share any part of themselves with us, we lose interest over time and give up on them. We build trust with that sweet spot in between. The exact pace will vary, as it will depend on your own individual experiences, but we are all capable of building trust.

A moment of bravery and vulnerability could be setting a boundary, eating when you're hungry rather than ignoring it, or allowing yourself to feel a feeling before doing anything with it (or suppressing it again).

Trustworthiness also means saying you're going to do something and then actually doing it. If a friend repeatedly tells you that they can meet at a certain time and then cancels or is late, you probably won't trust them to arrive on time, as they aren't displaying trustworthiness; they're saying they're going to do something and then aren't doing it. Similarly with yourself, say you're going to do something, then actually do it.

In order to build trust, we also need awareness. Interoceptive awareness is the ability to identify, access, understand and respond appropriately to patterns of internal signals. Build awareness first, then trust yourself to allow yourself to follow through and respond to that awareness and what your body is telling you that you need. Think of it as a sense, like touch or taste.

Notice what's going on in your body, build that awareness, then respond accordingly.

Hunger and fullness

We all have an innate ability to recognise when we're hungry and need to eat, and when we're full and it's time to stop. As babies, we are able to recognise our hunger and demand food, and when we're done we simply turn our head away. No one taught that baby when to stop eating. Unpolluted by diet culture, we are born to eat this way. But as we grow up, we may have layers of lessons and narratives pushed on us which stop us from accessing that. While it's not our fault that those are there, it is our responsibility to unwrap each layer, each unhelpful lesson, until what remains is our instinctive, intuitive knowledge of how much food we need.

One way we can do this is by noticing every 'should' that crops up in our mind around food and hunger. You might find it helpful to write these down as they appear in order to keep track of them. This could be, 'I should leave five hours between meals' (you really don't have to if you're hungry) or 'I should eat a salad for lunch' (why? Who is that coming from?).

Every time you hear a 'should', replace it with 'could'. 'I could leave five hours between meals ... but do I want to?' 'I could eat a salad for lunch ... but what are my other options?' See how a world of possibilities opens up.

Another way we can begin to access the core knowledge we

have around hunger and fullness is to practise consciously and deliberately noticing what our body is telling us. I like to use a tool called the 'hunger wheel'.* This tool (shown opposite) looks at hunger like a fuel gauge – with 0 on one side being totally empty and 10 on the other side being totally full. We can broadly divide these sections as follows: uncomfortable hunger (0–2), comfortable hunger (2–4), neither hungry nor full (4–6), comfortable fullness (6–8) and uncomfortable fullness (8–10).

Noticing hunger

There are three main areas of the body where we commonly notice hunger. Our stomach is the obvious one, where we might feel a sense of emptiness, or rumbling sounds that get louder and more uncomfortable. In our head we may experience a lack of concentration, an irritability (hanger – the combination of hunger and anger – is real), or maybe even just thinking about food a bit more. In our whole body we can feel a sense of tiredness or a lack of energy that might be contributing to hunger. I find it's worth starting with the stomach, as that tends to be the clearest for people, and go from there to other parts of the body.

What exact sensations we feel in each section is personal to us; for example, some people find their stomach starts making sounds when they're just a little hungry, whereas for others they have to be ravenous before any rumbling occurs. There are some broad themes, such as that feeling of emptiness where your

---

* If you're not a fan of this version with the numbers, you can find a version in the 'Resources' section of my website which uses colour gradients, not numbers. You can also find a pdf version of the hunger wheel with numbers.

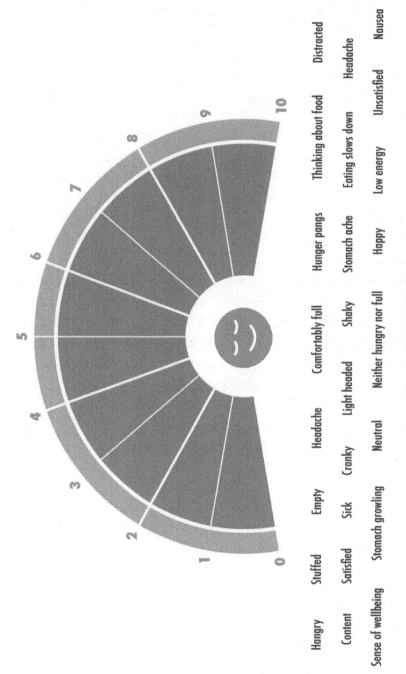

THE HUNGER AND SATISFACTION WHEEL

stomach is when experiencing comfortable hunger. Generally speaking, we want to spend most of our time in the comfortable areas of 2–8, in the same way that we want to drink water before we are so thirsty that we get a headache, or we want to go to the bathroom before our bladder is so full it hurts. Comfortable is where our body is happy and wants us to be.

If you don't experience any consistent hunger signals at all, this may be because you've been restricting for a long time and your body has, in simple terms, given up on sending those signals. By eating regularly and consistently, and keeping an eye out for them, they will return.*

I encourage you to write on this wheel, or make a copy on fresh paper, and take a moment to notice what the different sections feel like for you. What do you experience in your body when you're ravenously hungry? Slightly hungry? Not hungry or full? Comfortably full? Painfully full? You'll see that there are some words sitting underneath the wheel; these are guides in case you're struggling to find the right language to describe what's going on for you. You do not have to use them; they are simply there in case they fit for you. Remember: no one can tell you that your answers are right or wrong, because no one else knows what it's like to live in your body.

If you're used to spending a lot of time in painful hunger and fullness territory, you might be unsure about how gentle hunger and comfortable fullness feel. That's OK, you can leave those sections blank until you figure it out. If you have

---

* If you're in recovery from a restrictive eating disorder, it may be that you need to spend some time simply eating enough food to weight restore, with a focus on recognising and responding to hunger signals only entering the picture much later in recovery. It's important that you speak to your team about this.

spent a lot of time ignoring hunger, you might be at a place now where you don't notice it until it's an intense feeling, and it'll take time to rediscover what gentle hunger feels like. Start by making a note of the time when you start to notice your hunger. Let's say, for example, your hunger pretty consistently kicks in very suddenly and strongly at 1pm. From about 11am onwards, set an alarm or a reminder that's visible for you (I'm a fan of calendar reminders that pop up) every twenty minutes. Each time that reminder appears, stop what you're doing and take a minute to look inwards. Notice what's going on in your body. Through this deliberate practice you'll find that you begin to notice the subtle signals that weren't obvious before. Over time, this will become easier and easier, and you'll experience the benefit of having that extra awareness, as it allows you the time and space to make food decisions, rather than experiencing a frantic, desperate urge to eat something *right this second*.

Hunger v. thirst

'But what if I'm actually thirsty?' Hunger and thirst are two different things. We may struggle to differentiate between them due to alexithymia (explained in Chapter 8), or we may doubt our ability to tell the difference due to the influence of diet culture, but when we are attuned to our body we know the difference. We know it in the same way that we know the difference between needing a number 1 and a number 2. You can tell, right? Yes, sometimes you may need both, but even then you can tell that it's both. When diet tips say to drink water if you think you're hungry, that's utter garbage. If you're hungry, eat. If you're thirsty, drink. Use the hunger wheel to help you tell the difference.

Practise noticing

The whole purpose of the hunger wheel is to have a visual aid to help you practise interoceptive awareness in a deliberate and conscious way – it is not meant to be used forever. In that way it's like scaffolding: it gives you structure and support while you're building a trusting relationship with your body, but eventually it's taken down when it's no longer needed.

It's important to remember that some of what we perceive as emotional eating might actually simply be eating in response to physical hunger. I say this as I have often noticed that those individuals who regularly diet may feel that 'I can't possibly have been hungry so that must have been emotional eating' or 'that felt out of control and now I feel guilty so it must have been emotional eating', so it's a form of retrospectively assigning a negative emotional component to an eating experience.

Sometimes we eat quickly and seemingly 'out of control' because we are just so hungry. When you reach an intense form of hunger, feeling 'too hungry', this intense need can kick in where you feel like you just need food right now. This is a common experience when you're overly hungry.

To go back to the hunger wheel, when you go into the 0–2 territory of intense hunger, you start eating quickly and a lot, and you don't really notice the experience of gradually moving across the wheel to the fullness side, until suddenly you stop and think 'Whoa! I'm full!' Now you've gone past comfortable fullness into uncomfortable and even painful territory, and that's often where the guilt sets in, because it feels as if you've eaten 'too much' and it hasn't felt like a choice.

This is why I recommend trying where possible to eat when at around a 3 on the scale. It's the sweet spot that isn't too hungry so that your hanger kicks in, and it is hungry enough that food tastes really good and the eating experience is enjoyable. It also allows you to eat more slowly and more mindfully so that you can ideally recognise comfortable fullness more easily.

When I give clients the hunger wheel we always start with hunger and hunger only. We don't touch fullness until much later. The reason for this is that starting with fullness can feel like you're trying to eat less, so it can feel like restriction. By starting with hunger, we start with encouraging eating and noticing when it may be a good time to start cooking or start eating. It's not about restriction, as there's also no 'rule' that you can only eat when you're hungry. You can eat whenever you want for whatever reason you want. It's your body. But we want it to be a choice where possible, so you feel that you're in the driving seat of your life's decisions around food.

Recognising fullness

Once you feel like you have a good awareness of what hunger feels like for you, and you feel able to respond to it effectively, it's time to move on to fullness, and recognising the point of comfortable fullness with the aim of stopping eating around there. This is not coming from a place of restriction – this isn't about not being allowed to eat more, but more about feeling comfortable in your body.

When we understand what different stages of hunger and fullness feel like to us, we can then use this tool to begin to link food experiences to fullness; for example, you might be someone who needs plenty of carbs in a meal to feel really nicely full for several hours. Or you may be someone who finds they need plenty of protein to feel satisfied. Our needs and preferences vary, and it's about looking inward to find out what feels good *for you*, not anyone else. Fullness and satisfaction are slightly different things. You can feel full simply based on quantity of food, but satisfaction really comes from an enjoyment of the meal. Satisfaction can come from adding condiments, or from including a variety of textures, or from seasoning food well, or from having something sweet at the end of a meal, or from the cooking method (for me, roasting vegetables brings me greater satisfaction than boiling them, every time). Again, it's about what brings you satisfaction, and only you can figure that out for yourself.

One final point in favour of the hunger wheel: when we recognise and understand what our hunger feels like, it allows us to ask ourselves the question, 'Am I hungry or am I feeling something?' when we're staring at the fridge for the third time that hour. Familiarity with our own hunger signals allows us to more easily figure out the answer. Feeling hungry? Great, go and eat something knowing that you're responding to a physical need from your body. Not feeling hungry? Interesting... maybe something else is going on. Perhaps you're feeling something. In the next chapter, we'll help you work out what that is.

15

Feel Your Feelings

We've explored interoceptive awareness, and how to notice what's going on in your body around hunger and fullness. The next question becomes: what are you feeling?

Enter the wheel of emotions, shown overleaf. This is a tool to help work out what it is you're feeling. Emotions can appear deceptively complex, yet they are often surprisingly simple once we familiarise ourselves with them. If you have trouble recognising what you're feeling, if you are trying to unlearn lessons and judgements about your emotions such as 'sadness is a waste of time', or you tend to use vague words such as 'weird' or 'bad' to describe how you feel, this tool can be a helpful starting point.

What are you feeling right now? To work that out, start in the centre of the wheel, with the core emotions such as anger and sadness. These are helpful words to start with, and sometimes we need to be more specific; for example, there is a significant difference between feeling joyful and feeling hopeful, although these can both be forms of happiness. I encourage you to start at the centre, and at least try to get to the second ring of words to describe how you're feeling. Being more specific helps you to really understand what's going on for you and what you might

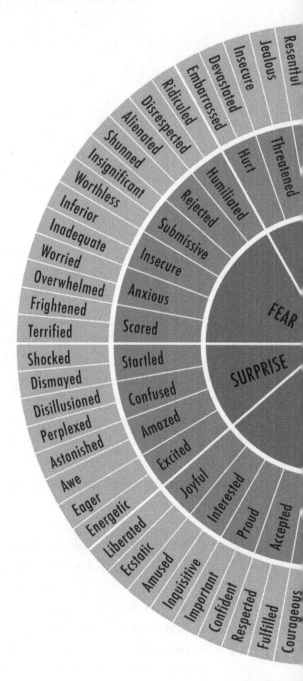

WHEEL

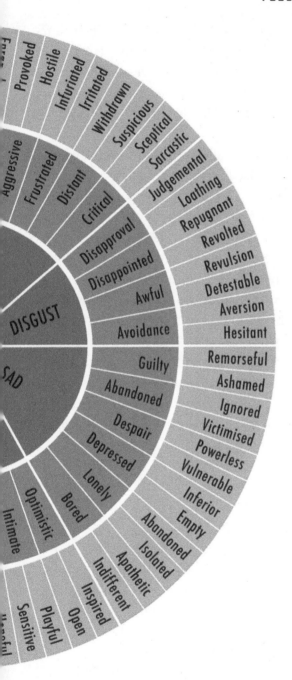

OTIONS

need. When you say you feel 'weird', what do you really mean? Do you mean uncomfortable? Vulnerable? Insecure? Hurt?

It may then also be worth trying to notice where these emotions live in your body. For many of us, anxiety can sit in our chest or in our gut. Sadness may be in our throat, while despair crushes our whole core.

Some of this originates in the fight-or-flight response, where acute stress causes an increased heart rate, dilated pupils and muscle activation. Some of it also links to the gut–brain axis: our two-way communication between the brain and the gut that helps to explain why we get 'butterflies' in our stomach (technically in our gut) when we feel nervous. But it goes beyond this – researchers have mapped which locations in the body are activated when we feel certain emotions, and the patterns are surprisingly consistent between people.[36] For example: we feel anger in our chest and arms, rising up to our face; happiness fills our entire body from top to toe; sadness sits in our chest, while also numbing our arms and legs; and disgust lodges in our throat. Although we don't fully understand why, our bodies can help us to identify and understand what we're feeling, especially when we're struggling to find the words.

What do our feelings tell us?

Now you know what you're feeling, you can hopefully more easily work out what you need to help with that emotion, whether that's solving a problem it's telling you about or finding ways to release and express that emotion. When we turn to food, it can be helpful in the moment by distracting us or temporarily allowing us to avoid that emotion.

To be an emotional eater is to be human, but an over-reliance on this one coping mechanism creates a fragile system.

Well-meaning advice from those who don't understand is usually to eliminate these foods from your vicinity. The cliché 'out of sight out of mind' has often already been tried and tested by the people I see and found wanting. When someone comes to my clinic describing emotional eating, they often say that they feel greedy, ashamed and out of control. I see it differently. What I see is someone who has found a coping mechanism that works, and who struggles when it's taken away. Food is the solution to an underlying problem. I see it this way: if you injure your leg, you may need crutches to help you walk while your leg heals. Now imagine if we took away your one reliable crutch: your food. You would probably have trouble walking, and the healing process would take so much longer. So I propose that instead of taking away food, your one dependable crutch, let's add several more options so that you have choice. Your trusty, reliable crutch, your food, is still there, but it's no longer the only thing you depend on. It's a much more stable and sustainable system.

When we add crutches or coping mechanisms it's important that we remember that not all crutches work for all emotions. For me, journaling can help when I feel sad, but it does fuck all when I'm angry. For me, and many people I speak to, anger has to be discharged physically, through kinetic energy. This stems from anger's physiological connection to aggression. When you become angry your muscles begin to tense. Inside your brain, neurotransmitter chemicals known as catecholamines are released which cause you to experience a burst of energy lasting up to several minutes, which is why there is an immediate urge to take action. At the same time, your heart rate accelerates, your blood pressure rises, your rate of breathing increases, and adrenaline rushes around your body preparing you in case you need to fight to protect yourself. When we take a few breaths instead of acting immediately, it allows us to engage our rational brain to consider a productive release for that anger.

This could be going for a walk, doing a boxing class, releasing a primal guttural sound, or scribbling on a piece of paper until it breaks, then scrunching it up and throwing it away. This way we recognise anger, take responsibility for it, and navigate it constructively, without hurting ourselves or anyone else. Then we can figure out if problem solving is needed.

Find out what does and what doesn't work for you

I always recommend trying a new coping mechanism while telling yourself that food is a backup option and *meaning* it. It's no good telling yourself that you can turn to food as a backup if you don't follow through with it – that's not exactly building trust, and it will make the whole process so much harder. Turning to food is not a sign of failure. It's simply a sign that food is what you needed, that the new coping mechanism isn't right for you, or that it isn't quite effective enough today; for example, one of my clients told me a story about how she eats canned potatoes when she misses her grandma because they serve as a reminder of her. That's a beautiful and wonderful thing, and food is absolutely the most helpful option in this case. Finding new crutches and coping mechanisms is an experiment. You start with a hypothesis: 'does journaling help me with anxiety?' Then you test it out. If the answer is yes, it does help, great! Add it to the list. If it doesn't, great! Now you know more than you did before. Knowing what doesn't work is just as useful as knowing what does work. It all takes you a step closer to understanding yourself better.

None of these crutches are replacements for food. They are in addition to food.

I encourage you to write down these lists, especially if you find you struggle to think clearly when emotions are strong (an understandable response). Placing this list in a convenient spot where you can access it easily may then help you find it, pick one item from the list, and give it a try. You have to find what crutches and coping mechanisms work for you, but here are a few suggestions from me to get you started. Give them a try, note what does and doesn't work for you.

Anxiety: Journaling, breath work, focusing on what is true. This last one is helpful if you find yourself lost in a 'what if' spiral of possibilities. By focusing on what *is true*, rather than what *could be*, it helps you to ground yourself in reality rather than being swept away by anxiety. Remember: you don't know what others are thinking or feeling unless they tell you.

Anger: Walking, exercise, scribbling on paper, releasing guttural sounds, venting.

Sadness: Crying, watching/listening to something to help release tears, journaling, curling up into a ball with a blanket.

Loneliness: Calling someone, giving yourself a hug, cooking something that reminds you of people you love.

Sometimes these crutches are short-term solutions, and that's all we need to allow the emotion to be discharged or to let it pass. At other times, finding and utilising a short-term crutch helps to give us the time and headspace to look into longer-term solutions. If you feel lonely, cooking a meal that reminds you of a loved one is great for taking care of yourself in the moment, and it then gives you the space to find a longer-term solution, such as finding a way to surround yourself with more people you care about. If you're feeling angry about an injustice at work, a boxing class can help to release that anger, allowing you to think more clearly about a longer-term solution, such as making a complaint or finding a new job. As we've also discussed, there could be deeper underlying problems, like a sense of purposelessness or a lack of self-worth.

Why am I doing this? What do I need?

The overall aim of finding new crutches is to ask ourselves important questions around food and emotions. When your self-critical voice says 'Ugh, why am I doing this?' (as a rhetorical question), I instead encourage you to ask, 'Hmm, why am I doing this?' with curiosity, and then answer that question. In a nutshell, what are you really hungry for? What do you actually need? What is the problem that food and eating is trying to solve for you? Sometimes food will still be the answer. At other times it will be food and another crutch. And at still other times it'll be something completely separate from food that helps.

Hopefully, by now you know which emotions are likely to be a trigger for you and why, thanks to the reflection you've done on previous chapters. Depending on what lessons you were taught as a child, and what beliefs you currently hold about your emotions now, finding new crutches for certain emotions means reshaping your relationship with those emotions.

Exploring these topics can elicit strong and overwhelming emotional responses. Sometimes these are emotions we've pushed down and avoided for a long time, either by comfort eating or by avoiding eating, and feeling them again is challenging. Ideally, we want to work towards being able to sit with our feelings before acting on them to allow ourselves the experience of simply feeling whatever it is we're feeling, to prepare for times when we are unable to act immediately. It also teaches us that these emotions aren't bad or wrong, that they can take up space in our bodies, and they don't immediately have to be discharged.

Carla, who struggled with an eating disorder and alexithymia, was doing really well in recovery and connecting to her emotions more, until one day it all proved too much, and she found herself returning to old self-harm behaviours in an attempt to manage the distressing emotions that were coming up. This happened when she sat quietly with her feelings after a lengthy period of being very busy, which left a backlog of feelings and hurt that suddenly rushed up and overwhelmed her. Her story serves as a reminder that it's important to take our time with our emotions – little and often is a helpful approach to take – and it shows just how strong our emotions can be when we feel ill-equipped to handle them.

If you're not there yet, that's OK! It can take time and practice to be able to sit with uncomfortable feelings, or feelings that we've been taught we're not supposed to feel and express. This is why we start with adding crutches first and learn to sit with feelings later.

How to sit with your feelings

Sitting with our emotions simply means allowing yourself to feel them, resisting the urge to get rid of the pain and not judging ourselves for having these emotions. It is the sweet spot between avoiding our feelings and wallowing in them. When we avoid, we may eat, and when we wallow, we dwell, we fixate, we ruminate, and we trigger secondary emotions such as guilt or frustration in a delicious spiral of self-flagellation. Neither approach is helpful. Sitting with our feelings means noticing them, naming them, accepting them and not judging them.

This process is not always an easy one. When we start to

release those emotions that are stored in our body from all those years, it can bring up painful memories and emotions so strong that they feel overwhelming. When I asked one of my clients to try sitting quietly instead of frantically cleaning and eating until she felt sick, she returned the following week with a story about an ex-partner who she had depended on for validation, and who had made her feel worthless. These were emotions and experiences she had avoided for years, and it was painful for her; after we had discussed them over several weeks she said she felt relief and was able to be kinder towards herself now that she understood herself better.

Sitting with your feelings – in practice

It sounds oh so simple and yet sitting with your feelings is deceptively challenging.

1. Find a comfortable spot to sit, without too much background noise. Try to minimise any possible distractions, so no music, no podcasts, no TV on in the background.
2. Close your eyes or lower your gaze to the floor. Breathe. Focus on breathing in and out slowly for a few moments, and then let your breath settle while you notice what comes up.
3. If you notice your mind start to focus on everything you need to do that day, that's fine, just bring yourself back with the question, 'What do I notice?' It may take you a few minutes to settle into it, especially if you're not used to sitting quietly, so take your time and be patient.
4. Don't analyse, don't try to figure out why something is coming up, just stay with it for now and experience it. Think

of it like birdwatching: you're not trying to count the birds or figure out why they're in your garden, you're just observing them and naming them without judgement.

Sitting with our feelings is so hard because our default evolutionary programming is to avoid pain and suffering for our own safety. This is helpful when there is physical pain we can escape from, but it is not always helpful when it comes to emotional pain. Of course, there are always exceptions; if a friend, family member or partner causes us pain through emotional abuse and manipulation, avoiding that person is absolutely helpful and protective. But when it comes to feelings within us like anger or sadness, feelings that we've been taught in life to avoid or not express, being able to sit with those gives us a sense of peace and agency that's so incredibly valuable. Life runs smoother when you recognise and work with your emotions, rather than engaging in an exhausting daily battle with them. Most clients who come to see me are looking for a greater sense of contentment in life, and this is one way I help them find it.

As I sit with my feelings right now, I can notice that my stomach is full (I'm writing this just after lunch), my legs feel a little restless as I've been sitting down all day, and after a minute or so I can feel some anxiety bubbling away in my chest. The accompanying thoughts I notice are about whether I'll get all my writing done on time and how much longer I can write before I have a train to catch later today. There's also a bit of sadness that I recognise I feel every time I have to leave my cat alone for a few hours. In just a few minutes, I'm noticing my thoughts, my feelings and body sensations.

I know the emotions I feel right now – the sadness and the anxiety – are fleeting. The anxiety will pass once I'm no longer writing, and the sadness will pass when I'm focused on my train journey rather than the beautiful cat I'm leaving behind. These emotions feel manageable. That's not always the case. If you sit quietly and your emotions feel overwhelming, as if they're crushing you or swallowing you or are simply larger than you, there's an additional step you might like to take: an anchoring technique.* This anchoring (or grounding) doesn't make the emotions go away, but it does help to place them in context.

Anchoring technique

1. Find a comfortable seated position and close your eyes. Take a few long breaths.
2. Notice what emotion is coming up for you. Name it, notice what it looks and feels like. Is it still or moving? Is it at the surface or right at your core? What words would you use to describe it? Perhaps place your hand where it lives in your body.
3. Notice that feeling, and now become aware of your body *around* the feeling. Notice how your body surrounds that feeling, your body that you can move and control. Perhaps move your body a little by stretching or rolling your shoulders.
4. Now notice this feeling, your body surrounding that feeling, and the world surrounding your body. Open your eyes and notice what you can see, hear and smell around you.

Notice how we haven't tried to make the emotion go away, but hopefully it's not so overwhelming anymore because we've located it within your body, so it can't possibly be bigger than you.

---

* You can find a recording of this anchoring exercise on my website.

This process only takes two to three minutes, and yet it can do so much for putting intense emotions into perspective and giving them less power over you. You haven't changed the emotion or removed it, but you *have* changed your perception of it to be more accurate. It's not bigger than you; it can't be, because it lives inside your body.

Emotions have purpose

Fighting or pushing away your emotions is such a tiring process, like trying to keep an inflatable ball under water. It will keep bobbing up when you're distracted or you get tired; it won't just go away because you want it to. Emotions move on when we work with them, accept them, process them, discharge them. Imagine not having to put in all that effort and energy anymore, imagine being free from that. Doesn't that sound like an amazing feeling?

Once you've sat with your feelings, you may find that just like clouds on a sunny day, they move on when they're ready, and they move on more easily than if you try to force them to go. Any process of acceptance, including around our emotions, is like those automatic doors on cars. If you press the button and patiently wait, they will close at their own pace. But if you try to force them to close, they stop moving and the whole process takes so much longer than it needs to. You may also find that these emotions are lingering, in which case you can turn to your list of crutches and coping mechanisms to help you out. Your emotions are what make you human, they will always be a part of you, so maybe it's time to stop fighting them and embrace them instead. After all, they're all there for a reason, and we can more easily figure out what that reason is if we recognise what's going on and approach it without judgement.

Sitting with your feelings, inviting them in and being curious about them helps to remove judgements that you have about them, and it helps you feel that you're working with them instead, so you're on the same side. Your emotions aren't trying to hurt you, they're trying to help you, and they all serve a purpose. In this way, a belief such a 'sadness is a waste of time' can transform into 'sadness is telling me that I need something or I care deeply about something'. 'Anger is bad' can transform into 'My anger is valid, and I can navigate it in a safe way that doesn't hurt me or anyone else.' These new beliefs are helpful, non-judgemental and validating.

First, we sit with the feelings, then we do something with them. First be, then do.

16

Countering Shame

Shame thrives in secrecy, and secrecy encourages shame. It's a horrible cycle that goes round and round and eats away at us, corroding our joy. This emotion, which Jungian analysts have labelled 'the swampland of the soul', makes us feel as if we are worthless.

There is a fundamental difference between guilt and shame, and it's important that we separate these to avoid any confusion or merging of the two. Guilt says, 'I made a mistake' – it's based on an action or a behaviour. Shame says, 'I am a bad person' – it's based on who you are at your core. This is what makes guilt so productive and helps us to behave better towards others, whereas shame eats away at us and becomes toxic.

When we feel shame, it's as though a spotlight is shone on all the dark, ugly parts of ourselves. Our instinct when it comes to shame is to hide what we are ashamed of, and that hiding is what messes with us more than the shame itself. If we're ashamed of our feelings, our urge is to hide our feelings. If we're ashamed of our body, our urge is to hide our body. If we're ashamed of our experiences in life, we feel a need to keep our experiences a secret from others.

Breaking the cycle

We break this cycle of shame and secrecy with openness, vulnerability and empathy.

This is a hard ask, because if there is shame there is usually a fear of judgement by others, and a fear that the shame will be reinforced. Usually, we have this fear because we have very real past experiences of being judged, or because we judge ourselves in the very way we fear others will judge us. Bringing shame out into the open is an act of bravery, because there is a very real risk of being hurt. There is an element of the unknown. If you knew exactly what was going to happen, there would be no bravery involved. There would be no risk. It would be easy.

Right now you may be thinking: *Well,* logically, *I know this person won't judge me, but I'm still afraid.* That tells me that even though you can think rationally about it, you don't believe this at your core. This usually results from your own judgements and experiences, and it has very little to do with the other person. It comes from within you, and it will not change until you are brave. All the logic in the world can't overpower fear. Shame is too powerful for logic. You have to accept the risk, accept the fear, and do the thing anyway.

You can bring secret eating out into the open in two ways. You can tell someone that you eat in secret; for example, by telling them that you wait for them to leave before having dessert or that you grab seconds from dinner after they've gone to bed. Or you can choose to eat those foods that you would usually eat in secret openly around others, by having dessert while they're still there, for example. Either works, it simply depends on what you feel more comfortable with, and what feels more manageable for you.

When it comes to shame around your body, I recommend

opening up to someone about your feelings and your experiences as a starting point. You don't even have to use the word 'shame' – I know some people really don't like it, and that's OK. You can simply tell someone you trust, 'I'm not feeling great about my body at the moment. I'm not looking for solutions from you, I just want you to listen and be a good friend.' If they respond in a deflective way by saying things such as 'But your body is great, you should love yourself!' Take a deep breath, and tell them, 'I appreciate what you're saying and I know your intention is to be helpful. But the reality is, I don't feel that way. And it's hard for me to even say that to you.' If they don't listen to what you need and continue to tell you how you should be feeling, perhaps consider discussing this with someone else.

Hopefully, what will happen when you do this is that you receive warmth and non-judgemental empathy from people. This is the most powerful response that's most likely to put a crack in the shame–secrecy cycle. Even if what you receive is that person not really giving a shit that you're eating chocolate in front of them, that is still valuable, as they are communicating to you that this is no big deal for them, not even worth commenting on. *They aren't fazed.* Maybe that can help you see for yourself that this can be no big deal for you too.

Bodies have value

We can reduce the shame we feel about our bodies by learning to see that our bodies have inherent worth and value no matter their shape or size. We can act in ways that are consistent with that belief, by wearing clothes that fit comfortably, not apologising for our body, feeding ourselves enough food, eating a variety of food, moving our body in a way that feels good, experiencing the pleasure of orgasm, moisturising after a shower, and accepting compliments from others. I always like to tell my clients: you don't have to agree with a compliment to accept it; you just have to accept that this person is being honest and showing you kindness. Rather than saying, 'Oh, this shirt is so old, I probably should have ironed it better', why not say, 'Thank you, that's really kind of you to say.'

If starting with food feels hard, and I understand if that's the case, I recommend buying some new clothes and immediately ripping out the label so that you can't focus on the size. Put those clothes on, close your eyes, and notice how your body *feels* in them, not how it looks. Are you comfortable? Doesn't it feel amazing? One of the smallest yet most powerful things we can do to feel more at ease in our body is to choose underwear that fits so beautifully that you barely even notice it. Every time you wear something that doesn't fit right, you can feel where it digs in, it heightens feeling self-conscious and it focuses your attention on all the areas of your body you aren't happy with. It distracts you from the more important things in life.

Alongside all this, we can also focus on what our body can do, and be grateful for what it allows us to do in life. We can broaden our definition of beauty to beyond what society and diet culture says is beautiful and acceptable. We can surround ourselves with people who accept our bodies rather than judge. The opposite of body shame isn't body love – it's body acceptance. The society we live in will never tell us that we are good enough, because it's not profitable. Accepting your body, warts and all, is a quiet act of rebellion. You don't have to love someone or something to accept them. Acceptance is not complacency nor is it a weary resignation. Self and body acceptance has, at its core, a drive to grow and a willingness to face the truth. This starts with acknowledging where you are now, even if it's uncomfortable.

Body acceptance

In the previous chapter we discussed sitting with your feelings, and I recommend doing the same with your body. Sit with your body and notice what comes up for you. Look at yourself in the mirror and just notice the thoughts and feelings that float to the surface.

Once you know where you are now, you can figure out where you want to go, and how to get there. If body acceptance is a goal for you, whether it's for the purpose of removing body shame or any other reason, I have an activity for you. It's one of my favourite pieces of homework to give clients.

Embodying acceptance

Imagine you're the star of the *Truman Show* or *Big Brother*, with cameras everywhere so that people can see you and hear you. They can observe your behaviours and what you say, but they have no idea what's going on inside your head; they don't have access to your internal thoughts and feelings. On two separate pages I want you to write down:

1. Everything people would see and hear that would show them that you feel insecure, shame or dislike towards your body.
2. Everything people would see and hear that would show them you accept your body.
3. Remember: no thoughts or feelings. How would you spend your time? What would you be wearing? How would you carry yourself? What would you be eating and drinking?

➡

> Who would you be spending time with? What would you talk about?
>
> 4. Note all the differences between the first and the second list. Each week, pick one or two items from the second list and put those into action. Over time, you will gradually embody that person who does accept themselves and their body fully, even if you're not quite there on the inside.

People who accept their bodies automatically treat their bodies more kindly, whether that's by eating in a way that feels good for their body, moving their body in a way that feels good, keeping up with healthcare appointments, spending time outside, or all of the above. In the end, body acceptance means reaching a place where your body takes a back seat, and you don't think about it that much at all, because it's not the most valuable or the most interesting thing about you. It's what that body enables you to do that counts most, whether that's to earn a degree, run a marathon, birth a child, hug a friend, or change the world. Body acceptance, and therefore spending less time thinking about your body, frees up your time and headspace for far more important endeavours. (In Chapter 19, Overcoming Defences, I give some more exercises to help you to start the process of accepting your body.)

Shame and blame for the past

Of course, we don't just feel shame around our food and bodies, we may also feel shame around our life experiences, especially if deep down we blame ourselves for what happened to us. Self-blame is common, especially with childhood trauma, as a way for the brain to cope, and shame will nestle comfortably alongside that blame, taking up space and refusing to move. But it has to move. Maybe here is where you can speak to a therapist to work through your blame and shame. Maybe you need to forgive yourself for doing what you had to in order to survive. Maybe you need to accept that you were powerless, it wasn't your fault, and there's nothing to forgive yourself for. In my experience, therapy is the best place to talk this through, because a therapist is there to listen, be honest with you and offer you empathy in a non-judgemental way. I can tell you it wasn't your fault until the end of time, but you have to reach a place where you believe it yourself.

If you're still unsure about therapy and want to engage in some personal self-reflection first, then I invite you to consider this question: what do you gain from believing it was your fault? I recognise that this can be a deeply uncomfortable question, and yet the answer is key to understanding what is blocking you from moving into acceptance. If your immediate answer is, 'I gain nothing', I can tell you with absolute certainty that you're wrong. There is always a pay-off. For many of us, blaming ourselves allows us to believe that there was something we could have done, that we had some control. But that's just not true. I don't care if you were drunk, I don't care what you were wearing, I don't care if you argued back; that does not make you culpable. You are not to blame for someone else's decision to take advantage of your vulnerability. Everyone has the right to be vulnerable *and* safe.

Regardless of where your shame lies, there are big steps and small steps you can take to dismantle it. Sometimes bold, brave moves are needed, like being open about secret eating. At other times, smaller but still bold steps can provide a kind of systematic desensitisation to shame. Daisy's case is a good example of these smaller actions. She felt that she was bigger than her friends and felt self-conscious and ashamed of her body around others. She judged herself and her body so harshly that she also feared others would do the same. We came up with small steps together that could help her to gradually confront her fear, experience lack of judgement and reduce her shame. One week she wore shorts, another week she spent less time sucking her stomach in around others, the week after she wore spaghetti straps, all building up towards wearing a bikini on holiday – which she did. The fear hadn't completely gone away, but she had built up enough experience of not being judged that she could get past it and enjoy herself.

It's also worth taking time to disentangle shame from guilt. If you made a mistake and tell yourself, 'I made a mistake, I'm such an idiot and a failure', maybe reframe it as 'I made a mistake, and that sucks.' Make it about what you did, not who you are. Guilt, not shame.

Shame is sticky and clings to us unless we actively take steps to wash it off. Now you have those steps in your arsenal, you can put them into action. Alongside everything I've already mentioned, the final step I want to offer you in countering shame is to practise self-compassion. This acts as a powerful remedy to shame, and it also carries so many other benefits with it.

17

Finding Your Self-Compassionate Voice

As we have seen, if your default position is to be hard on yourself, if your inner critic is loud, if you judge yourself harshly, if you use 'should' a lot, if you're a perfectionist, or if you carry a lot of shame and blame, you are distancing yourself from a better relationship with food and yourself.

If you have a strong inner critic, you're also more likely to experience problems such as depression, anxiety, deep shame, stress and overwhelm, feelings of helplessness, decreased motivation and body-image issues. A strong self-critical voice drives you towards disordered eating, not away from it.

Fortunately, I have several tools in my toolbox that I like to use to help take some of the power out of the self-critical voice, and to nurture the self-compassionate voice. I am slightly unconventional in my approach, as I like to offer strategies from several therapeutic modalities, some of which claim to be incompatible. My clinical experience tells me that offering you all these means that you can find the one that is right for you. I encourage you to try them all.

Being kind and understanding – to yourself

Instead of ruthlessly judging and criticising yourself for various shortcomings or flaws, self-compassion means being kind and understanding when confronted with your personal failings. We all have flaws and inadequacies; none of us is perfect.

In a nutshell, self-compassion is showing yourself kindness and care, in the same way that you would a friend. Often the way we talk to ourselves is incredibly harsh, and we use words that we would never dream of saying to someone we care about. We somehow think that we are the exception to the rule. I want to be very clear that self-compassion is not coddling or letting yourself off the hook when you messed up. It's not self-indulgence. It's not lying to yourself. Self-indulgence tells you that it's OK to spend an extra few hours in bed – you can make up the work tomorrow. Self-criticism tells you that you're lazy and useless. Self-compassion notices that your body needs some extra rest, but places a reasonable time limit on it so that you can still be productive. When it comes to food, self-indulgence might look like ordering a takeaway five nights in a row because it's easier than cooking. Self-criticism tells you that you're being greedy and beats you up for even ordering a single takeaway. Self-compassion recognises the value and self-care of cooking something at home that's delicious and satisfying, even if you'd rather stay on the sofa.

Self-compassion does not say 'it's OK' when it's not OK. It's honesty and truthfulness with kindness rather than judgement.

Kristin Neff is an associate professor of psychology in the US and has been credited with conducting the first academic studies into self-compassion. She defines self-compassion as having three elements:

1 **Self-kindness** means being warm and understanding towards ourselves when we suffer, fail or feel inadequate, rather than ignoring our pain or whipping ourselves with self-criticism. The reality is that we will fail, we will make mistakes, things don't always work out the way we want them to, and our worth doesn't change as a result of that. We still deserve to be treated with kindness rather than criticism.

2 **Common humanity** Suffering is part of being human, and we are not alone in our suffering. It is not something that happens uniquely to us but to everyone, and recognising that we are vulnerable and imperfect – just like everyone else – creates a sense of shared experience rather than isolation.

3 **Mindfulness** is a non-judgemental state of noticing what we feel and think, without trying to push any of that away or down. We cannot ignore our pain and feel compassion for it at the same time. We don't want to avoid our pain, but we also don't want to become overly attached to it and wallow in it either. You'll notice how this ties in nicely with our earlier discussion on sitting with feelings (on page 155).

When we bring these three components together in the way we talk to ourselves, we offer ourselves self-compassion. Say you fail an exam or apply for a job and get rejected. Your default might be to say to yourself, 'You failed, you're such an idiot. You're going to sit here and work on this day and night until you get it right.' It's critical and punishing and cruel. You would never (I hope) say this to a friend or family member. When we incorporate the three elements of self-compassion, we might instead say, 'That didn't work out at all the way I wanted, and that hurts (mindfulness). This happens to people all the time, I'm not alone in this (common humanity), and I can work hard on this tomorrow after a good sleep to try to do better (self-kindness).' Notice how this doesn't deny the reality of what happened and what you feel.

Talking to yourself with compassion might feel uncomfortable at first. *Good*. That means you need it. It's uncomfortable because it's unfamiliar, and it's treating yourself as though your self-worth is high and fixed in place, which may be at odds with your beliefs about yourself. Stay with that discomfort, understand why it's there, and keep going.

Another way you can practise self-compassion is by writing a letter to yourself from the perspective of a future version of yourself who loves themself (and therefore you) unconditionally. It allows you to place yourself in the headspace of a version of you who is already where you want to be, and has the wisdom of hindsight to offer the current-you their perspective and guidance. How would you talk to yourself? What do you wish someone would say to you now? What do you need to hear right now, today? Is it encouragement? Forgiveness? Hope? When I wrote my first letter like this, I started it by saying, 'Dear Pixie, you're amazing. It's time to stop being so hard on yourself, because your life will get so much better when you do.' Both the writing and the reading of this letter can be an incredibly powerful experience that can start to change how you view yourself, speak to yourself and treat yourself.

If letter writing isn't for you, that's OK, perhaps you can start with reframing your self-critical thoughts. Some people find it helpful to write them down when they appear, to really build awareness of how often they appear or what exact wording is used. Externalising these criticisms and judgements onto paper (or the notes app on your phone) totally changes the way you perceive them. I've often heard from clients that the very words they write down seem so harsh once they read them back to themselves and they're no longer contained in their mind.

Challenging automatic negative thoughts with CBT

If you've ever even caught a whiff of cognitive behavioural therapy (CBT) you may have heard of the concept of ANTs: automatic negative thoughts. These are unhelpful or irrational thoughts that pop into your head without your control, often in response to a trigger of some sort. Because they're automatic they can seemingly come out of nowhere, and we may not even pay attention to them properly, but they can have a negative impact on how we view ourselves and the world; however, with time and effort, we can identify them and reshape them into something more positive.

For example, the trigger for the automatic negative thought may be saying something that a friend openly disagrees with. The ANT may be, 'I messed up, I'm such a bad friend, they probably hate me and think I'm an idiot.' An alternate or adaptive thought could be, 'It's OK to disagree with friends. It doesn't mean they think badly of me, it's interesting to hear different points of view.'

When we directly challenge and reframe our automatic negative thoughts, it can help us, over time, to reduce their frequency and have the positive thoughts become more automatic. It's only by repeatedly, consciously changing these thoughts that we eventually get to a place where this happens automatically. It's like learning to drive a car; at first each move you make requires conscious effort. Then, the more you practise, the more natural it becomes, until eventually you can drive while talking to someone without any difficulty. Thoughts are not that different.

Replacing automatic negative thoughts (ANTs)

If you want to give this a try, find a piece of paper, place it landscape, and split it into three columns with the headers: 'trigger', 'automatic negative thought' and 'alternate/adaptive thought'. Then, whenever you notice an ANT appear, write it down and identify the trigger if you can. You can usually identify what the trigger is by noticing what happened just before the thought appeared. If you don't have time in the moment to come up with an alternate thought, that's OK, you can always write it in later. Repeat until you notice your thoughts changing in the moment.

Here's an example:

Noting your ANTs		
Trigger	**ANT**	**Alternative/adaptive thought**
Ate dinner and felt painfully full after.	'I'm greedy, I ate too much.'	'I ate past comfortable fullness, and it hurts, but it doesn't change my worth as a person.'
A friend told me that something I said hurt them.	'I'm such a bad person. How could I do this to a friend?'	'I'm grateful that my friend felt they could tell me this. I apologised, and I'm going to learn from it.'
I made a mistake at work, and someone pointed it out.	'I'm such an idiot, I'm a failure, and everyone knows it now.'	'Everyone makes mistakes, I'm allowed to make mistakes too.'

Defusion through ACT

In CBT we challenge our negative thoughts about ourselves, we dissect them and we provide counter-arguments. This can be an extremely helpful approach, but it is far from the only approach. We can also use the skill of defusion, which is a method from acceptance and commitment therapy (ACT).

Fusion occurs when we feel that we *are* our thoughts and feelings – we are fused together. We see this in our language when we say 'I am anxious' rather than 'I feel anxious'. Fusion is inherently harmful, so if it's not harmful, it's not fusion. We wouldn't bother defusing from thoughts and feelings that we are settled and comfortable with.

There are six main types of fusion, which all interweave and overlap:

1. Fusion with the past (for example, rumination).
2. Fusion with the future (for example, 'what if' spirals, catastrophising).
3. Fusion with self-concept (for example, 'I am broken').
4. Fusion with reasons (for example. 'I can't change because people won't like me').
5. Fusion with rules (for example, use of 'should' – 'I shouldn't get takeaways').
6. Fusion with judgements (for example, 'I'm being an idiot').

You'll know if you're fused with a thought, or hooked by it, because the thought will have incredible power over you. A tell-tale sign that you might benefit from defusion is if you feel you are overwhelmed by, lost in, wallowing in, consumed by, or controlled by, your thoughts and feelings. Defusing from our thoughts allows us the space to focus on other things that might be more important to us in life, rather than being trapped in a cycle of rumination.

My favourite way to practise defusion is simply by adding, 'I'm having the thought that ...' to whatever sort of thought comes to me. It's so simple and effective. Just notice the difference between these two statements:

'I'm not good enough.'

v.

'I'm having the thought that I'm not good enough.'

Amazing, right? The first one is spoken as an absolute fact, whereas the second one is a thought. It doesn't remove it or avoid it, but it recognises it for what it truly is: a thought, not a fact. It takes some of the power out and allows us to take a step back and go, 'Ah, I see what this is: it's a thought I'm having, that's interesting.' It allows us to notice rather than being engulfed by it. If you want to take it a step further, you can say, 'I'm noticing that I'm having the thought that ...' for some extra distance and unhooking.

If you're a kinetic learner (you prefer to learn through movement), try saying the first statement with your hand right up close against your face. That's what it feels like when you're hooked by the thought. It's right up in your face and it's hard to see anything else in the room, or even the words you're reading here. Now place your hand at arm's length while you say the second statement, the defused one. It's still there, it's taking up some of your attention, but you have perspective because you can see the rest of the room around it clearly.

It doesn't even matter if the thoughts are true or not. That's what is so great about defusion – assessing the veracity of your thoughts is not the point. We're not here to debate whether you are or aren't good enough – that's a conversation for another time. The aim is to help you unhook from that thought in that moment, to allow you to see it for the thought (not fact) that it really is, and have enough perspective to get on with your day rather than feeling stuck.

Find what works for you

In my clinical practice, I always try to offer my clients several options, because some of these tools are more suited to certain people than to others, and some are more applicable for certain types of thoughts or situations than others. Let me give you an example. Poppy was diagnosed with cancer at a young age, and after it was successfully treated, she developed orthorexia to try to take some control over her body, and out of a deep fear of the cancer returning. She was seeing a CBT therapist while also seeing me, and in one of our sessions she confided in me that she felt it wasn't working for her. She was doing the homework, she was challenging her negative and self-critical thoughts that made it hard for her to eat certain foods, but she wasn't making any progress. The reason being, her fear-based, self-critical voice would say, 'but what if you get cancer again?' That argument always won, and I can totally see why. Of course it would! How can you argue with cancer? So we dropped the CBT strategies and turned to defusion instead. It worked a treat and helped her to reach a much happier place with food that was more relaxed, more flexible and more enjoyable.

Some people find that arguing with their own thoughts suits them really well, and they find the practice useful because they feel that they're fighting for themselves. Others find the challenge tiring and unhelpful, and instead they prefer to create some distance from their thoughts. In my view, everyone could do with a little more self-compassion in their lives, and practising speaking kindly to themselves. Self-criticism isn't working for you, otherwise you'd keep doing it and you wouldn't be searching for solutions in this book. Talking to yourself more kindly and unhooking from your thoughts brings you closer to a positive relationship with food – and with yourself.

18

Adaptive Perfectionism

When we spoke about perfectionism in Chapter 9, I made the distinction between adaptive and maladaptive perfectionism, with a focus on the latter. Now it's time for us to turn to the more helpful side of perfectionism.

Unlike maladaptive perfectionism, which is characterised by unrealistically high standards and harsh self-criticism, adaptive perfectionism is healthy, as it relates to having ambition, a drive to succeed and being goal-oriented. Adaptively perfectionistic individuals set high but realistic standards, and they don't resort to harsh self-criticism when these standards are not reached.

If you've identified yourself as a maladaptive perfectionist, all hope is not lost. It is completely possible to transform this into a more healthy, adaptive perfectionism that allows you to have a more fulfilled life. We can do this by challenging perfectionistic thinking and behaviour.

Perfectionistic thinking

The thought patterns behind maladaptive perfectionism are typically: self-criticism, all-or-nothing thinking, repeatedly using 'should' and 'must', and fear of failure. We can tackle all these.

We've already discussed the self-critical voice and ways to cultivate a self-compassionate voice in the previous chapter, so if you're a perfectionist you will find great benefit in combining those skills with the techniques that we'll go through in this chapter.

All-or-nothing thinking, or black-and-white thinking, has a notable absence of any middle ground or grey area. A reminder that if you're someone who says 'Fuck it!' when one thing doesn't go right, if you use 'always' and 'never' a lot when it's not *actually* true, or if anything below an A is a failure, you're a classic black-and-white thinker. The easiest way to reshape black-and-white thinking into grey is through language. Notice when you hear yourself saying 'always' and try saying 'sometimes' or 'often'. Notice when you say 'never' and try saying 'rarely'. Notice how differently it sounds when you say, 'I always get this wrong' compared to 'I sometimes get this wrong.' The latter sounds much gentler, more realistic and more encouraging to me. I can pick myself up again after that and try again, because it feels that there's a possibility of succeeding.

A close relative of all-or-nothing thinking is catastrophising, where your mind immediately takes you to the worst-case scenario. It's not the same as over-exaggerating, because you're not doing it intentionally, your mind goes there automatically. In my clinical practice I often see that perfectionists with anxieties around food and their body tend towards catastrophising, as the thought of any deviation from food rules or deviation from dieting immediately brings up the 'but what if I ...' worst-case scenarios. My response is usually, 'But what if something else happens?'

Finding alternative options

If black-and-white thinking or catastrophising have you locked into only two outcomes or possibilities, as an exercise it could be worth writing down as many other options as you can imagine, the more the better. For those who love logic and writing, this can be a helpful task.

Maladaptive perfectionists I speak to are often also people-pleasers (as explained in Boundaries, Chapter 11) and have a need to be a perfect friend. This can lead them to engage in another type of unhelpful thinking called mind reading. If a friend cancels on you and you automatically assume that means they hate you, then this is you. This is a tough one to shake; it generally forms because you have been taught, at some point in your life, that things are usually your fault. It's time to shake that assumption, and to train yourself to consider alternative possibilities. If your friend cancels, what else could be going on? Make a list and see how focusing on just one of those possibilities – the one where it's your fault – isn't accurate or helpful.

Writing exercises are so helpful for all these thinking styles that form part of maladaptive perfectionism, and we can take a similar approach with excessive use of the word 'should'. You may have noticed by now that I'm not a fan of this word at all, and most of us would benefit a great deal from using it a lot less. I often challenge my clients on their 'should' statements, so much so that they often start correcting themselves before long, which is a joy to witness. I recommend reframing 'should' into 'could'. 'Should' is expectation and pressure; 'could' is possibility. Alternatively, I suggest turning 'should' into 'want to' and seeing how that feels. Again, 'should' is expectation and is often external, whereas 'want to' is desire, it's internal. It comes from within you. Just turning a statement like, 'I should exercise more' into 'I want to exercise more', or 'I should be able to stop eating when I'm full' into 'I want to stop eating when I'm full' is already a great start and a step in the right direction. Maladaptive perfectionism involves 'should' and unrelenting pressure; adaptive perfectionism is all about 'could' and a drive to do well.

If you connected with several or all of these unhelpful thinking styles, you might want to combine all these writing exercises into one: a thought journal. In CBT this is known as the 'ABC' model, which stands for Activating event, Beliefs and Consequences'. While this is similar to the ANT table we explored in the previous chapter, this one specifically focuses on identifying unhelpful thoughts and thinking styles that are associated with perfectionism. It looks something like this:

How the ABC model works			
Activating event (trigger)	Beliefs and thoughts	Consequences	Unhelpful thinking style
What was happening at the time?	*What were you saying to yourself?*	*How did you feel as a result? What did you do?*	*Were these thoughts catastrophising? All-or-nothing thinking? Mind reading? Using 'should'?*
My jeans didn't fit.	*'I should fit into these jeans.' 'I'm useless.'*	*Frustrated, sad, annoyed. Almost cancelled my plans.*	*'Should' All-or-nothing thinking*

Sometimes we need to take some time to familiarise ourselves with what is actually happening in our brains and what patterns our thoughts have before we can do meaningful work to change this. A thought journal helps you to identify your triggers, forces you to notice how you're talking to yourself, and then allows you to combine this with self-compassion work to change. That's how you turn your maladaptive perfectionism into a more adaptive form – one thought at a time.

High standards and failure

A lot of us have a tricky relationship with failure. Fear of failure can be linked to many causes and can often have its roots in childhood, where you may have been routinely undermined or humiliated by parents, teachers or other significant adults.

Maladaptive perfectionists often have a high fear of failure and a very low bar for what constitutes failure, such as getting a B rather than actually failing an exam. Perfectionists also often equate mistakes with failure, which means, ironically, that you're more likely to experience failure as a perfectionist than as a non-perfectionist. On top of that, in order to try to avoid failure, perfectionists often procrastinate, because you can't fail if you don't even try.

In my own experience of developing more adaptive per-fectionism, creating a more helpful relationship with failure involved practising failure and sitting with the discomfort of it, and also changing my perception of failures I've experienced in life; for example, I failed to achieve a place at medical school twice despite having the correct grades, and while it was dev-astating at the time, it turned out that it was easily one of the best things that has happened to me. If I hadn't failed there, I wouldn't have ended up in the job I created for myself, after I spontaneously applied to study nutrition just two months before the start date. Failure is inevitable in life, so we might as well apply the perspective of trying to learn something from it when it does happen.

The idea of 'practising failure' seems like a strange one, but it makes sense: if you can demystify failure, become more comfortable and familiar with it, it will steadily lose its power over you. You have to figure out what this looks like for you based on your own understanding of yourself. It could be stumbling over your words and not apologising, wearing clothes that don't quite match, going outside without make-up, answering a question in class/at work when you're unsure if you have the right answer, asking for help with something (as this means admitting that you can't do it perfectly alone), or trying a new hobby and sucking at it in front of other people.

I also recommend telling people you trust about your failures. Speaking from personal experience, it is a profoundly healing experience when you reveal your failures to someone and they say, 'Same!' Hearing about other people's failures is also helpful, but you have to join in with your own.

'Good enough' is good enough

Ideally, we don't want to aim for 'perfect'; we want to aim for 'good enough'. Good enough is good enough. It may be worth considering, instead of trying to do something perfectly, what would it look like to do a 'good enough' job. Implementing the principle of 'good enough' does not mean deliberately aiming to do low-quality work or to be careless. Instead, it means clearly identifying what good enough means in your particular circumstances, based on the outcomes of your work and what you're hoping to achieve. This will vary in different scenarios, and in some cases your standard for good enough might end up still being quite high. In other cases, however, it might mean that you can ease off, not fail, and have a better quality of life. My trajectory with this over the course of three qualifications has been fascinating for me to look back on. When I studied biochemistry, I was firmly rooted in my maladaptive perfectionism, and as such nothing less than perfection was good enough for me. I was only happy if I was top of the class, which I achieved, but at the cost of my personal life. When I studied nutrition, I still had high standards, but now I didn't care how well I did compared to others as long as I achieved the highest grade: a distinction. I had started to move towards a more adaptive way of approaching my studies, and had so much more fun as a result. Finally, in my counselling and psychotherapy qualification I had moved squarely into adaptive perfectionism, as I had done a lot of self-exploration and also realised along the way that no one actually cares what your final grade is as long as you pass. So, my new 'good enough' became passing the course, working hard without sacrificing my well-being, and enjoying the process. My grades for individual assignments have ranged from a pass to a distinction, and everything in between. The world didn't end, and I'm better off for it. What does good enough look like for you? Perhaps it's:

- Aiming to cook at least four nights per week rather than demanding that you never order a takeaway.
- Checking over your work twice rather than ten times in case there's a single error.
- Having a designated cleaning day rather than keeping everything spotless 24/7.
- Delegating tasks rather than staying late trying to do everything yourself.
- Writing for half an hour rather than expecting yourself to write an entire essay in one go.
- Asking for help and advice rather than trying to do it all alone.

- Aiming to exercise for twenty minutes a few times per week rather than expecting yourself to always do a full hour.
- Choosing clothes you feel comfortable in today rather than emptying your closet to find the perfect outfit.

In a nutshell, developing more adaptive perfectionism looks like this:

- Noticing your unhelpful thinking patterns and actively changing them.
- Re-evaluating your relationship with failure by making friends with it, so that it becomes less frightening.
- Setting yourself standards that are 'good enough', not perfect.
- Celebrating when you succeed at something or do well. If you don't meet your standards, evaluate why, see if they're still too high, and practise self-compassion.
- Practising over and over again until you notice change.

When we reshape our perfectionistic thoughts and behaviours into something more adaptive, we reduce our risk of anxiety and depression, we're less likely to procrastinate, and we're more likely to live a life we actually enjoy. Because isn't that the point in the end? Beating yourself up for not having a 'perfect' body, or not getting 'perfect' grades, or not eating 'perfectly' hasn't helped you get to where you want to be in life. Let go. Choose 'good enough'.

19

Overcoming Defences

As we learned in Chapter 7, we all have defence mechanisms, because they arise out of a need to protect ourselves. Although they do a great job at it, they can often outstay their welcome and prevent us from growing, or from seeking out the help and support that we need in order to grow. The fact that you are reading this book tells me that your defence mechanisms are not impervious, and that at the very least there are moments of doubt in your mind. Even if you're in a place of acknowledging that there are issues you want to resolve for yourself, denial can creep in when the going gets tough.

Working towards overcoming denial

Denial can take many forms: saying 'I'm fine' when we're clearly not; avoiding seeking help for something so that we can convince ourselves that it's not important; minimising our experiences and trauma in life; rationalising and coming up with excuses to justify ourselves; blaming others for something that is our responsibility.

Denial is powerful, because it is there to try to help us. But avoiding our emotions, our memories and our experiences can lead to unintended consequences. Everything you push down eventually comes back up. In the meantime, it sits and ferments away inside you, until the pressure becomes too much to handle. It's worth letting it out when you are prepared and know what's happening.

In practice, this means working with what comes up on a regular basis, rather than delaying and delaying until you're forced to confront it. It's like having to pay your tax bill once a year instead of in your monthly payslips – trust me, as a self-employed person, it *hurts*.

When it comes to someone's relationship with food, a form of denial I often see is around choice: the perception that everything we eat is something we've chosen to eat. Although I don't ascribe to the idea that you're powerless in the face of your disordered or emotional eating, I think acknowledging that it doesn't *feel* like a real choice is important. As I often say to my clients, 'if you were really making a choice, I don't think you'd choose this'. What we call 'choices' can be so deeply ingrained that they become unconscious. Your automatic thought isn't a choice, but countering that thought is. Your emotions aren't a choice, but how you express them is. Your trauma responses aren't a choice, but understanding them is.

Working towards overcoming defence mechanisms such as denial can take many forms. Writing and journaling is one of my favourites, as it can help you to confront and admit what's happening in your life once you see it written down in your own words. When a client says, 'I can be hard on myself sometimes, but it's not that bad', writing down their self-critical thoughts in a day can open their eyes to the reality. Beyond journaling, mindfulness can allow you to take a step back and notice what's going on and assess before reacting, whereas a good therapist can help you hold up a mirror to yourself and see what's really there. The other advantage of a therapist is that they can challenge you in the moment and smash denial right when it comes out of your mouth. When Roger tells me, 'What happened to me wasn't that bad', I have a good enough relationship with him that I can tell him to just *stop it*. If needed, we can go over questions that we've talked through before. These are questions I encourage you to ask yourself as well if you've experienced anything that could be described as traumatic in life:

'What do you gain from minimising your experiences?' Perhaps it means that you don't have to think about them or talk about them, or even pretend they didn't happen. Maybe it means you can try to convince yourself that your childhood was OK or your parents were actually good parents.

'What would it mean for you if what happened to you was a big deal?' Maybe it means you were powerless and there was nothing you could do, and feeling powerless is deeply uncomfortable. Perhaps it means that your whole bubble of denial is shattered and you have to face the pain of that.

'If a friend told you this story, would you say that it's not that bad?' I bet you wouldn't.

If you're a fan of visualisation, I'd like you to close your eyes and imagine yourself floating inside a bubble. This is your bubble of denial. What thoughts, beliefs and narratives live inside this bubble and maintain it. How do you feel towards these narratives? Do they feel cosy and comforting? Now picture the space outside that bubble. What does the landscape look like? What thoughts, beliefs and emotions live out there for you? If those feel frightening or overwhelming, come back to your bubble. With time, you can increase your exposure to the world outside your bubble of denial, until eventually the bubble pops because it can no longer sustain itself.

If you're still sitting there telling yourself it's not a big deal, ask yourself:

- If it's not a big deal, why do you feel the need to keep it a secret?
- If it's not a big deal, why do you feel shame?
- If it's not a big deal, why is it bringing up distressing emotions and memories for you?

It *is* a big deal. Time to break out of denial, and move towards acceptance.

Reaching acceptance

Many years ago, I rolled my eyes at the idea of acceptance. I associated it with giving up, until my therapist sat me down and talked it through with me. He was very convincing. I'm a big fan of acceptance now.

Acceptance is freedom and it is peace. It's the moment I realised that I could talk about my father's death without feeling an intense wave of sadness. Acceptance does not mean liking, wanting, choosing or supporting. It means being at peace with the reality of what is, and ending the suffering of battling and denial. It's not a passive process; it's active.

- You may need to accept your body as being outside the standard beauty ideal.
- You may need to accept that your parents weren't good parents.
- You may need to accept that your emotional eating is your brain trying to help you.
- You may need to accept that you're using your body as an excuse not to find love.
- You may need to accept that diets just don't work for you.

- You may need to accept that you're holding yourself back out of fear.
- You may need to accept that the friendships, relationships or family dynamics you're in aren't working for you and it's time to get out.
- You may need to accept that you're not OK.

The stages of grief

Whatever you need to accept, this is your sign to start doing it.

As we have discussed before, there are several stages of grief that sit between denial and acceptance, although we can experience them in any order. Alongside these two there's also despair, bargaining and anger. Which one of these is coming up for you right now as you read this?

Is it denial? Are you telling yourself, 'This doesn't apply to me', when you know deep down it does?

Is it despair? Are you feeling sad, lonely, vulnerable or empty right now?

Is it bargaining? Are you using 'what if . . .' or 'if only . . .' statements to get out of staying with this?

Is it anger? Are you feeling irritated at me right now for bringing this up? Are you resenting reading this?

You may experience several or all of these as you work towards a place of acceptance. I'm not going to sit here and tell you that it's a journey full of rainbows and sunshine; it's painful. But there are small ways that you can begin to practise it right now.

To give you an example, if you're working towards accepting that dieting doesn't work for you, your denial might show up as your brain just saying 'Nope! Dieting *will* work for me!' Your anger may say, 'How dare Pixie suggest diets don't work.' You may then want to bargain, saying, 'But what if the next diet we go on *does* work?' The thought of that may then bring up sadness, as you begin to process how much time you've wasted on dieting. You may cycle through this a few times before reaching that place of quiet acceptance that dieting isn't for you.

Practising acceptance around difficult and traumatic experiences you've had in life that have shaped your relationship with food and yourself can start with simply staying with all the emotions that come up for you around this topic, allowing them to exist for a while, and then moving on from them. Accepting your emotions means spending time with them, just like we've spoken about several times already.

Practising acceptance after emotional eating or overeating can look like telling yourself, 'I feel uncomfortably full – it doesn't feel good. I'm going to try to learn from this and move on', and then moving on. Acceptance means not punishing yourself afterwards by restricting or being cruel to yourself, because it doesn't help, it just produces a cycle of restricting and overeating round and round with guilt fuelling the fire. Acceptance means moving on and listening to what your body needs, including rest if appropriate, and returning to a normal, regular eating routine the next day.

As we have already seen, something that many people find tricky to accept in their lives is their body. Reaching a place of body acceptance doesn't mean loving yourself every second of every day, nor does it mean you're happy with all of you and that you don't want to change anything. It means seeing your body, recognising yourself, showing kindness to your body, and just being OK with it right now in this moment with no strings attached. No 'I can only accept my body when it's a certain size' nonsense. As I explained in Chapter 16, Countering Shame, body acceptance is by definition *unconditional*, meaning that you accept your body regardless of size, weight, ability, age, or any other factor.

Start the process of accepting your body

Body acceptance isn't reached in one big swoop. It's through your small everyday interactions with your body that you show acceptance – the way you touch your body, dress your body, talk about it with others, even look at it in the mirror. Here are some examples of how you can begin that process for yourself:

- Write a thank you letter to your body outlining what amazing things it's done for you, whether that's to run, hug a friend, give birth, or simply keep you alive for all these years. Include an apology if you feel you have something to apologise for.
- Touch your body with kindness. No more pinching and prodding, just gentle touch. You could do this by really noticing how it feels to moisturise your body after a shower. Give yourself some orgasms too while you're at it.
- If you are able-bodied, perhaps you can cultivate some gratitude for what your body has enabled you to do; for example, my arms let me cuddle my cat today, while my legs enabled me to go for a walk outside while it was still sunny.
- Practise body attunement by asking yourself, 'What is my body telling me?' A body-scan meditation can help you check in here, as well as practising recognising

and responding to hunger and fullness cues. You can follow a guided meditation through an app, or simply take a few moments to breathe slowly, close your eyes and scan your body from top to bottom, noticing anything that comes up.

- Buy clothes that fit. Your body will thank you for it and you'll feel more comfortable living in your body.
- Accept compliments from others. Remember: you don't have to agree with what they're saying; you're simply acknowledging that they're saying something kind. I promise you, over time, it will feel less strange, and you will start to believe that you are a person who is deserving of compliments.
- Familiarise yourself with your reflection. You can't fully accept yourself if you don't know what's there to accept. If it feels uncomfortable, try starting by looking at yourself in the mirror while brushing your teeth.
- Recognise that the purpose of your body is not to look good, but to contain your amazing brain and to help you achieve what you want in life. Your body is one of the least interesting things about you as a person. This is also where we can ask those beautiful and deep existential questions like 'What are my values?' and 'How do I define myself?'

Try starting with one of these, then add more as time goes by until you're building up an arsenal of tools to help you reach a place of acceptance. It's not an easy process – there are billion-pound industries out there desperately trying to convince you that your body is flawed and not good enough so that they can sell you the solution.

※

Self-acceptance, whether it's around who you are, your body or what you've experienced in life, is a challenge. A challenge that's made even harder when the world around us tells us that we are not OK or that we are not good enough. It is harder to accept your body when it does not conform to what society tells us a body 'should' look like and when you have to face fatphobia and weight stigma on a regular basis. Accepting your identity as an LGBTQ+ person is tough when we face the threat of homophobia. Systems of oppression, whether racism, fatphobia, homophobia or ableism, or an intersection of these, make the internal process of acceptance more of a battle than it should be. But it is not impossible.

For many of us, self-acceptance is a lifelong journey that has to adapt to all the shit life throws at us, and all the changes that come with ageing and growing as a person. That may sound daunting but it's also beautiful: as humans we are never a 'finished product', we are constantly evolving into a new version of ourselves.

20

Setting Boundaries

When we first looked at boundaries in Chapter 11, we explored how setting boundaries can be beneficial, but that other people can initially be resistant to our requests. Now it's time to explore different ways in which we can develop effective boundaries to free us from the constant messages and judgements that we might receive about weight and our body.

If you're a people-pleaser or have grown up believing you have to be responsible for managing other people's emotions as well as your own, setting boundaries is going to feel a little scary.

Boundaries are hard. We can never predict how somebody else is going to respond to us setting a boundary. If the people around you aren't used to you setting boundaries with them, they will likely be surprised and may perceive it as a personal attack, or take offence. That's OK. Just because people expect you to have no boundaries or weak boundaries, it doesn't mean you have to keep catering to that.

In order to set boundaries, you need to know what you want. In previous chapters we've discussed swapping 'should' for 'could' or 'want', and that same exercise can help you tap into what boundaries you need to set based on your wants and desires. If you're struggling to articulate where you need boundaries, or what you want to change about situations that leave you feeling upset and uncomfortable, consider first writing down or clarifying what you want. In fact, I recommend making a note of both what you want, and what you don't want, so that you can clarify both what you're moving away from and what you're aiming towards; for example, you can combine: 'I don't want people to comment on my food when we're eating' with 'I want more varied and interesting conversations at the dinner table.' Or you can pair a desire: 'I want my child to grow up with positive body image' with a boundary: 'I don't want my family to comment on my child's weight in front of her.' Now you have both a boundary and an intention.

Setting boundaries can look like saying no, putting yourself first, breaking out of competitive diet-focused friendships, or communicating clearly how you like to be treated. I'm a big believer in preparing and practising for these kinds of scenarios so that you can build the confidence to say it when the situation demands it. I'm going to offer you a couple of scenarios, examples and possible responses you might get and how to handle them. Consider these templates to get the ball rolling and to help you find your own words that fit for you.

Saying no

'No' is a complete sentence. It's a cliché, but it is true. No is often an uncomfortable word to use on its own. If someone offers me something that I don't want, I will happily say, 'No thanks, I'm fine.' If someone makes plans and invites me, I may respond, 'Thanks for the invite, but I'm afraid I can't make it', or 'Sadly, that doesn't work for me.' Notice how these responses would generally be described as polite, and that I haven't given a reason or justification for not attending. You don't owe anyone an explanation if you don't want to give one. I have even been known to say, 'Sorry I have other plans that day', when those plans have been to sit on the sofa and watch Netflix, because I'm an introvert and know my limits when it comes to social interaction. It's true, I do have other plans; the fact that they don't involve other people is nobody's business except mine. I don't feel a need to explain myself to others because it's not up for discussion or debate.

As a healthcare professional, I regularly find myself in positions where people want to tell me about their diet or their 'food sins', and people love asking me what I think about various diet/wellness charlatans, books, documentaries and so on. I also often get asked to do my job for free. I've been to the dentist where, mouth wide open, I've been asked what I recommend for bloating, or should my dentist try cutting out gluten? I love my job, but not this part, and I end up setting a lot of boundaries like this. 'No, I can't give you advice when I don't know you', 'No, I don't want to hear about your diet', 'No, I don't want to debate with you whether your sister healed her [insert condition] by cutting out [insert food here] or by following [insert diet here].' I say no a lot.

If you want to practise saying no, maybe start with messaging or typing, as that might feel easier to do – you can psyche yourself up, take a deep breath, and press send. But what if you get the dreaded, 'Oh no, how come?' reply? You have options. I like to go for the apologise-and-deflect strategy. 'I know, sorry! Maybe another time?' or, 'Yeah, sorry, I hope you have a wonderful time though!' That usually does the trick, and by that point it's usually clear that I don't intend to share my reasoning with them.

Food, diet and body talk

When you are in recovery from an eating disorder, disordered eating, chronic dieting or body image concerns, it can be challenging to be surrounded by food and diet talk, whether it's at home, at work or with friends. You may have once been a contributor to these conversations, but now find them uncomfortable as your relationship with food has changed, and you don't want these thoughts to take up space in your mind. Now you have people around you talking about their diets, commenting on your food, making comments on your appearance or weight, and you don't want that. It's time to set some boundaries.

I find the simplest way to set this boundary is simply to say, 'Please stop commenting on my food/weight.' Clear and simple. Ideally, you receive a response acknowledging the boundary and respecting it, but of course people sometimes react defensively.

Defensive response: 'OK, no need to be so dramatic, it's not a big deal.'

Your reply: 'It might not be a big deal to you, and that's fine, but this is me telling you that it's important to me.'

Or:

Defensive response: 'I don't understand why this matters to you.'

Your reply: 'You don't need to understand it; I just need you to respect my wishes.'

Sometimes you may not feel comfortable setting a boundary with someone in the moment; for example, in a group setting, and would rather have that conversation later one to one. In those situations I find a simple deflection does the trick.

Comment: 'You've gained weight!'

Immediate deflection: 'I got a new sofa too.'

People don't expect this kind of deflection, especially if they're used to you (or people in general) taking the bait and engaging in conversation about your body, so social norms usually kick in here and people start talking about your new sofa instead.

Possible response: 'Yes that's lovely, but I'm concerned about you, you've gained weight, are you OK?'

I like to deflect again: 'I'm more concerned with this new sofa – doesn't it really bring the room together?'

In my experience, people give in after a second deflection to avoid any perceived awkwardness. As long as you present yourself as calm and confident, with a polite smile, you'll tend to direct the conversation successfully elsewhere.

Remember: if all else fails, you can always excuse yourself and go to the bathroom to escape and breathe for a few minutes. By the time you come back the conversation will likely have moved on. If diet talk is persistent around you, and it doesn't affect you too much, silence is also an acceptable tactic, by simply not joining in. People will notice your silence over time, and you get to protect yourself from engaging in a conversation that doesn't serve you. I have often heard from people that this feels like a safe starting point for them, as it feels like a more gradual progression from engaging in diet talk, to staying silent, to eventually speaking up and setting a boundary. It might even remind others that making unsolicited comments about people's body shape isn't acceptable, and that shaming someone won't magically change their body.

Unhelpful helping

People usually have good intentions, and they respond well when you recognise their good intentions. Keeping this in mind has helped me to set boundaries when receiving unsolicited advice; for example, 'I know you're trying to be helpful, but this actually isn't helping me', is my go-to response, as it acknowledges the good intention, but it makes it clear that their assumption about what's helpful for me is wrong. In my experience, although people can be taken aback in the moment, sometimes they are grateful to have a clearer idea of how to help in particular situations. The best-case scenario is that they ask, 'What do you need?' or 'How can I help?'

This highlights an important aspect of boundaries. It's not just about saying 'no' and telling people what not to do, it's about showing people how to treat you better and with the respect you deserve. It's an act of love and care that shows you are invested enough in a relationship with another person that you're willing to stand up for it, work on it, and draw attention to where there's room for improvement.

Emotional boundaries

One of the greatest lessons I ever learnt in life was around emotional boundaries, and knowing which emotions are mine and which belong to someone else. When we take on emotions from other people that don't belong to us we end up saddled with all this additional baggage that weighs us down. Our own emotions are our own responsibility, and they are enough for one person, we really don't need to be carrying more than that. I want to emphasise that this is not to discount empathy; if you are empathising with someone you are still feeling your own emotions, not someone else's.

There are two main reasons we end up with weak emotional boundaries in this way: firstly, because we have been taught in early life that it is our responsibility or even our duty to take on the burdens of others; secondly, because someone has inadvertently and (hopefully) unintentionally hit at an insecurity of ours.

Developing stronger emotional boundaries could also be described as not taking things personally when they're not about you. This begins as an internal process, by asking yourself, 'whose emotion is this?' If someone is loudly sharing about how they need to go to the gym after having such a large lunch, and you feel guilty, ashamed or suddenly uncomfortable in your body, what's going on there? Remind yourself that this person isn't talking about you, they're talking about themselves, and it is not your responsibility to take on their own disordered attitude towards food and exercise. What they are saying has *nothing to do with you at all*. It only becomes about you when you let it.

If in this situation you're thinking to yourself: *But if they're saying that about themselves what must they think about me and my body?*, pause and take a breath. Mind reading is a fruitless and thankless endeavour that will keep you spiralling into endless unspoken possibilities rather than anchoring you to what was actually said. Did this person actually say anything about you? No. Stop taking on their baggage, it's not yours.

Enough with the people-pleasing

If you're a people-pleaser, you will likely have experienced emotional dumping: people may have learned to expect and assume that you are always available to listen to their problems, because you consistently put other people first. They know you'll pick up the phone, put down your work, or reply to their message quickly and listen until they have finished dumping all their emotions on you. Being on the receiving end of this can be exhausting, especially if it happens often and without warning.

It's time to set some boundaries around this. If you have a friend who consistently emotionally dumps on you, you can write them a message saying something like, 'I really value you as a friend, and I want to be there to support you with what you're going through. I need you to ask me if I have the emotional capacity to listen right now, and I promise I will answer honestly.'

This requires both you and your friend/the other person to be in agreement about this. They have to take responsibility for asking the question, and you have to be responsible for answering honestly. If you always say yes, even when you mean no, the boundary is meaningless and nothing has changed. Your yes becomes infinitely more valuable when you are also able to say no.

Who is influencing you?

Boundaries are not simply about saying no or asking people to stop something, it is also around who has access to you. Another way to look at this might be: who has the power to influence you? Social media is the biggest culprit for this and also often the easiest one to change, as you can decide who you follow and what content you see. If you feel inadequate while you're scrolling through bikini shots and 'what I eat in a day' videos then ... stop. Unfollow and choose what you actually want to see instead. If you have old diet books in the house that you no longer want to be exposed to, donate them. If someone keeps commenting judgementally on your food pictures online, mute them. These are small things that will add up significantly when you consider how many times you walk past those books each day, or how much time you spend scrolling. These are small changes that set boundaries around who has access to you, and who is influencing you.

Setting boundaries requires you to be brave and vulnerable, which is challenging to do when you've been taught that your own needs come last, or that what you want is not important. Your needs *do* matter, you *do* deserve to put yourself first, and what you want *is* important. As with all things, the more you practise setting boundaries, the easier it becomes, and the better your life will be, because the people who stay in your life are the ones who respect you, not the ones who treat you like a pushover.

21

Building Identity and Meaning

When it comes to improving your relationship with food and your body, all the work we do boils down to one simple thing: when food and your body stop taking up so much headspace it allows you to focus on the more incredible and meaningful aspects of life. Without food occupying your every waking thought, without constantly being aware of your body, what more could you offer yourself and the world around you? Who could you become?

Many people who go on diets or develop disordered eating in adolescence don't get to experience the forging of identity in that psychosocial stage of life. Food obsession can easily become a key 'island' of identity, and going through the process of recovery and improving your relationship with food can feel like losing a significant part of your identity. That can feel really tough. It's one of the reasons why recovery is so hard – in some ways you have to find yourself again, so we need to find out what else there is to you as a person.

This doesn't just apply to those who are in recovery from food and body-image issues, it can also be relevant for people who divorce or are widowed after a decades-long marriage and have to find out who they are without their partner, people who go through a difficult break-up at a key moment in life, people who find out that they're adopted, and people who become unemployed or retire. Big changes in our life circumstances can be an opportunity to reflect and work out: 'Who am I without this person or thing that I've lost?'

The big, 'who am I?' question is an intimidating one, so rather than delve into it directly I'd like to take you on an identity journey. I like to think of identity as concentric circles, with the innermost circle being the absolute core of who you are, the most accurate and concise answer to the question of who you are. We start on the outside, and we gradually work our way in.

What do I have in life that matters?

I like to start by asking my clients, 'What do you have in your life?' An 'I have . . .' approach can feel more gentle than 'I am . . .', and it can help you to take stock of what you do already have in your life that's important to you. For me, I have a large collection of houseplants, and they help my house feel like a home. I have my work, my family, my cat . . . any number of things I can list that matter to me.

Make a list of everything you can think of, no matter how large or small. If it matters to you, write it down. Already you can probably identify some items on this list as being more important to you than others. How would you feel if these were taken away? Which can you live without? Which ones do you not appreciate as much as you feel you would like to?

How do I spend my time?

Following on from this, think about how you like to spend your time. What brings you joy? If you're struggling with this one because food or dieting has become your identity to the extent that everything else fell away, that's OK. When rediscovering identity, I find it can be helpful to look back to the proverbial 'before times' and how you spent your time then. What were you doing with your time that brought you joy before you developed an eating disorder, or were dieting, or had to work long hours, or had body-image issues that prevented you from engaging in activities that brought you joy? You don't have to go back to anything you don't want to or feel you have moved on from, but it can be a good place to start looking if you feel that food is all-consuming. Genevieve developed an eating disorder in her early teens, and when we met she had started and dropped three different university degree courses because she just couldn't work out what she wanted to do with her life. This was partly because she was engaging well in the recovery process and was feeling that keen loss of identity that came with that. She didn't know who she was anymore without her eating disorder. When I asked her what would bring her joy before her eating disorder, she mentioned horse riding, baking and going to the cinema. We made a plan for her to try re-engaging with these one at a time, to see which still brought her joy now. She was able to connect with all three and rediscovered a part of herself that had been lying dormant through all those years of restriction. Her pie chart of identity morphed from a solo eating-disorder slice with no real room for anything else to demolishing that to make way for a whole host of slices: a horse-riding slice, a cinema slice, a friendship slice and a fun slice. In this way, by going back to what used to be part of her life, we expanded her pie chart into something more varied and stronger.

What does your own pie chart look like in terms of what occupies your time? How does it compare to your ideal version? If you're not sure what that would look like, what could you try to explore to see if you want to include it in your pie chart?

What is my body's purpose?

This ties in very nicely with one of the components of positive body image: body purpose. In other words, 'What is my body's purpose beyond aesthetics?' My body allows me to embody my purpose in life, which is to help people through the work I do. It allows me to do that through my presence in the room, my voice, my reassuring smile and my gesticulations when I speak, and through my use of my connection with my body as an example with my clients. My body also allows me to hug and care for those closest to me, including my cat, as well as to travel around the world to experience new and exciting adventures. These all have very little to do with the way my body looks, which is exactly the point.

Your turn: what is your body's purpose beyond how it looks?

How would people I'm close to describe me?

Once we've explored all this, I then like to move on to the 'How would your friends describe you?' approach. You can ask them directly how they would describe you, as long as you believe what they say and don't doubt them. If you don't want to ask your friends, ask anyone you're close to who you trust would be honest and open with you.

Some people like to go so far as to write the eulogy that they would want to be read out at their funeral by a close friend or family member, which I'm aware could sound quite morbid, but it can actually help you to focus on the most important aspects that people are most likely to remember. This also has another added advantage in that people don't generally say a lot of negative things about someone at their funeral: any readings or reflections focus on positive traits and achievements, and it forces you to see yourself that way too.

Exploring yourself from this external perspective can help you to be kinder and more objective about yourself, rather than looking inwards through the smog-tinted glasses that is your self-critical voice. After all, there are very good reasons why people like you and choose to spend time with you. If you're still really struggling with this, ask your friends or a partner or anyone close to you to write something for you, then adapt it into your own words.

What are my values?

As we delve deeper and approach the core of who you are as a person, it's time to talk about values. Our core values tell us what matters most to us in life. These are personal and individual, and everyone will have a different opinion about what's most important. Values usually consist of a single word and can include kindness, honesty, growth, love, loyalty and compassion, as well as more concrete concepts such as family, friends and health.

Identifying your core values helps to clarify what is important to you, and it can act as a guide when you're unsure about a choice in life. When we live a life that is in accordance with our values, we are generally more content and we experience less distress. When we are living in a way that is at odds with our values, or far away from them, we can feel unsettled and discontent. By identifying what our values are, and whether we are following them in life, we can identify any areas for improvement and find ways to bridge any gaps, with the intention of making our lives better for ourselves.

If you'd like to give this a try, ask yourself, 'What do I value?' and consider the suggestions below. If you're unsure if something is a value, try saying, 'I value . . .' and see if it sounds right; for example: I value kindness, I value family.

Values

Accomplishment	Consistency	Freedom
Accountability	Creativity	Fun
Achievement	Dependability	Generosity
Adventure	Determination	Goals
Affection	Discipline	Goodness
Authenticity	Diversity	Growth
Balance	Efficiency	Hard work
Beauty	Empathy	Healing
Belonging	Enjoyment	Health
Career	Enthusiasm	Helping others
Caring	Equality	Honesty
Challenge	Ethics	Honour
Commitment	Exploration	Hope
Communication	Fairness	Humility
Community	Faith	Ideals
Compassion	Family	Independence
Competition	Fidelity	Ingenuity
Connection	Fitness	Insight
Consciousness	Focus	Intellect

Intuition	Prudence	Strength
Joy	Purpose	Teamwork
Justice	Reliability	Temperance
Leadership	Resilience	Thankfulness
Love	Resourcefulness	Thoughtfulness
Loyalty	Respect	Tolerance
Mastery	Restraint	Tradition
Merit	Satisfaction	Trust
Money	Security	Truth
Nature	Self-actualisation	Understanding
Openness	Selflessness	Uniqueness
Opportunity	Serenity	Vision
Optimism	Service	Vitality
Order	Spontaneity	
Preparation	Stability	

Take a quick look at the list above and cross out the least important ones for you until you've reduced it to ten. Try to do this without overthinking it. Rewrite this list of ten, then cross half out and reduce it to the five most important ones. Finally, bring it down to your three core values, the ones that are most important to you in life.

If you're unsure, ask yourself what you value about different aspects of your life; for example, what do I value in my work? I value money. What do I value about money? Opportunity. So opportunity stays while money can be crossed off. What do I value about my friendships? I value openness. And so on.

Try not to overthink, rationalise and introduce 'should' statements. Crossing something out doesn't mean that it doesn't matter to you at all. It simply means that it matters less than something else. There are no right or wrong answers; it's personal to you. These three core values are a part of your identity. In fact, I would argue that they're close to the core of who you are. In my experience, I will only share my core values with people I am close to, because it feels so integral to who I am, and I will always offer my clients the opportunity to not share theirs with me if they feel uncomfortable doing so.

Once you've identified your core values, the question becomes: are you living your life in accordance with these values? Consider this question in the context of your work or education, your leisure time, your relationships with others, and your relationship with yourself. That last one – yourself – is the one where many of us find that we're not living close to our values. You may show compassion at work, you may volunteer in your down time, you may be very compassionate towards family and friends, but what about compassion towards yourself? If you find that you are not living your life in accordance with these values, there is a great opportunity to bring yourself closer to them by showing yourself compassion. I have found this can be an incredibly powerful motivator for people who otherwise struggle with concepts such as self-compassion, self-kindness and self-love. Let's take another example: trust. If you don't trust yourself and your body, if you suppress your feelings and ignore your hunger signals, you are not living according to your core value of trust.

Of course, our values can change with time and the stage of life we're in. As a child you might value adventure and reliability, as a teenager you might value belonging and trust, as a parent you might value family and commitment, and later in life you might value communication and dependability. If you go through a period of great change and growth in life, it might be interesting to come back to the list of values and see where you end up this time. Change is part of being human, and that means our values change too.

What is the meaning of my life?

Forging meaning and discovering identity are often inter-linked. Through our understanding of ourselves and what matters most to us (our values) we can forge a reason for living our lives.

If you're a religious or spiritual person, do you believe that a higher power bestows your life with meaning? How do you go about searching for what this is for you? Meaning can be about religion and the connection to something bigger than yourself, which can bring incredible comfort, and it can also help to take you away from food and your body. I may not be religious myself, but I'm pretty sure that your chosen deity (or deities) hasn't decided that your life's purpose is to fixate on your weight, to be on a diet forever or to hate your body.

If you're more of an atheist, like me, meaning can be some-thing you decide to create from within. For me, my purpose in life and the meaning that I create in life is not something that is bestowed upon me, it's mine that I choose for myself. I find a huge sense of meaning in the work that I do, in facilitating changes in my clients that they desperately hope for. Meaning can be cultivated through relationships, a family, a sense of legacy, or leaving the world a better place than you found it.

What do you consider the meaning of your life to be right now? Regardless of which way your beliefs tend, it's a process of discovery and can also change with time. Your core values can help to guide you there.

Who am I?

So far we have asked ourselves:

- What do I have in life that matters to me?
- How do I spend my time?
- What is my body's purpose?
- How would people I'm close to describe me?
- What are my values?
- What is the meaning of my life?

When we bring together the answer to these questions, it brings us closer to answering that final question: who are you? It may not be a complete answer; some might argue that you can never have a complete answer to the question of identity, but it can absolutely be good enough to satisfy your needs. You understand the things that are important to you. Your pie chart will have several significant slices or be on its way there. You can feel a sense of purpose beyond how you look and what you eat. At the very least, your sense of identity will be broader and more varied than 'the dieting one' or 'the healthy one' or 'the person with the eating disorder', and with that comes a stronger foundation within yourself that leaves you less vulnerable to the influence of others.

This is where your true power lies. Not in your dress size, or in how much you ate today, but in what you are capable of, and how rich your life is once there is space for you to flourish. A healthier relationship with food is not the end goal. It is what you do with that which truly matters, and which will truly bring you joy.

Building a Healthy Relationship With Food

I help people build scaffolding.

The beautiful and bittersweet nature of the work I do, whether it's in my clinic or through this book, is that my presence is temporary. It has to be, otherwise I'm not doing my job properly. My role is to facilitate your growth and learning so that you can prepare yourself for a life where you can face the challenges thrown at you, and where all this becomes easier.

We may be coming to the end here, but really it is just the beginning.

To return to the people whose stories we've heard in the book, each one of them decided at some point that it was the right time to begin working towards a healthier relationship with food and themselves. That's not a process that can be rushed: they were ready when they were ready, and not before. Jemima was able to start dating again and no longer feels she needs to change her body to be worthy of love; Xena has been setting boundaries left, right and centre, and she still celebrates every time her boundaries are respected; Pietro now accepts himself fully; Carla no longer feels like a robot; Ethan is able to express anger effectively, although it's still scary sometimes; Roger has reached a point where he no longer believes what happened to him was his fault and he can notice and describe what he's feeling when asked; Hazel is starting to put herself first, which has not been without difficulties; and Lara has been able to find an identity beyond food and is thriving knowing who she is. All had different life experiences, all did the incredibly brave work of looking inwards, and all are in varying stages of recovery from disordered eating. I hope their stories have given you hope for yourself and your own relationship with food.

When enough is enough – towards change

We all have to start somewhere. Everyone I speak to, including you, has a moment where they decide they've had enough, that they want to pursue a better relationship with food and themselves. That moment is a powerful one. Look where it's taken you already.

There are a great many questions I've asked you to reflect on over the course of this book. I want to take some time to revisit the most important ones.

Where did you learn your relationship with food? Where did you learn your relationship with your body?
I have always found it is easier for us to be kind and compassionate towards ourselves when we have understanding. Now that you know what has shaped you into the person you are today, you can make more sense of your experiences, and see that there are very valid reasons why food might be hard for you, or why you've been on so many diets, or why you dislike your body so much. This level of self-awareness can be painful but illuminating.

The power of knowing that we have been taught to feel the

way we do about food and our bodies, the way we feel about ourselves as a whole, is that it means we can *unlearn and relearn*. You, as you are now, are not set in stone. No one is born hating themselves. No one is born with disordered eating. Now you know what you have learned, you can move forward with the unlearning.

What's stopping you from developing a greater relationship with food and your body?
If it were simple, if there were no barriers in your way, you would have done it by now. But there are barriers, and now you know what those are, you can begin the work of dismantling them so that they no longer hold you back.

What can you do to move towards the relationship with food and your body that you want?
What tools do you need in your toolkit to improve your relationship with food and your body? Which tools and skills that I have offered you will you try first? Which ones can you see presenting a real challenge?

You may find that before you can start exploring the hunger wheel (on page 144) you need to work on your perfectionism (Chapter 9) and self-compassionate voice (Chapter 17), so that you can approach interoceptive awareness (Chapter 14) with a greater level of kindness towards yourself.

You might find that you need to sit quietly with your feelings and become more skilled at staying with the discomfort before you can challenge yourself with any of the other tools available ('How to sit with your feelings', page 155).

It may be that you need to accept that the difficult experiences you've faced in life were not your fault, understand the ways in which they still significantly impact you today, process your shame (Chapter 16), and feel all the emotions that come up for you around this, before you even think about setting boundaries (Chapter 20).

What is your food story?

The answer to this question brings everything together, the past, the present and the possibilities for the future. What does your story look like so far? Where do you want it to take you? Can you see yourself doing what you need in order to get there? I recommend writing this out for yourself so that you can come back to it one day when you have grown into the relationship with yourself that you want, in order to remind yourself of how far you've come and how much it was worth it.

What I really want you to remember is this: having a healthy relationship with food doesn't mean you never eat for emotional reasons, you never skip a meal, you never eat something and regret it, or you never have a bad body-image day. All those things will happen, because you're human, but what will change is how often they happen, and how you respond when they do.

Having a healthy relationship with food and your body means eating in accordance with your hunger signals, and then sometimes eating when you're not hungry because you're bored or because someone has offered you something that looks delicious. It's stopping eating when you're full, and sometimes eating past that because the food is just so damn good. It's having a diverse range of coping mechanisms for your emotions, and sometimes using food to soothe because it feels good. It's feeling your feelings rather than suppressing them, and also recognising that sometimes you have work to do and your emotions have to wait until you're home and have time for them. It's talking to yourself kindly, and recognising when that self-critical voice still pops up anyway. It's knowing who you are, and also recognising that this will change over time. It's accepting your body for all the things it's done for you and will do for you, and also sometimes looking in the mirror and thinking 'Ugh, I look so bloated today.' It's standing firm in yourself and also allowing yourself to be influenced by the right people around you. It is all these things, because it is flexible, adaptable and based on a foundation of trust. Even if you never had that foundation, or you had it and then lost it, I believe it's never too late to build it for yourself.

Throughout all this, you can move away from thinking of emotions as good or bad, or bodies as good or bad, or foods as good or bad, and you can start to see the nuance and the grey in all these things. There is no such thing as a bad emotion, no such thing as a bad body, and no such thing as a bad food.

Of course, the advantage of being able to hold this book in your hands and place it on your shelf is that you can take it back down again and open it whenever you need it, and I encourage you to do so. Your relationships with food and your body are lifelong and ever changing, and there are times when you may need to revisit what you have learned, create a deliberate and conscious practice again, and remind yourself of what it feels like when you benefit from this. Because life is more meaningful when you process your traumatic experiences, your shame and diet culture; when you overcome your barriers; and when you have a toolkit of skills that allow you to look beyond food and your body.

Imagine all the things we'd get done if we weren't spending all that time and headspace thinking and worrying about food and how our bodies looked. Imagine how we could change the world. Promise me one thing: when these worries drift to the back of your mind and free up all that space, do something that matters. I don't care how big or small that something is. Make it count.

Postscript

Seeking Therapy or Nutrition Counselling

Having worked through this book, you might decide that you want to seek therapy or nutrition counselling. If so, this section will give you some guidance on how to proceed.

What kind of therapy is right for me?

There's no obvious answer to the above question, as it depends on what kind of person you are, what your concerns are, and how you like to approach self-development and self-awareness. It's important to remember, however, that the most important factor determining your success in therapy or nutrition counselling is the therapeutic relationship. In other words, do you like the professional you're working with? Do you trust them? Do you feel comfortable with them? Do you feel some kind of connection? If you answer yes, then you have a solid foundation that makes everything else easier. If the answer is no, then the process will be so much harder, sometimes even impossible. Finding the right professional is like dating: sometimes the right person for you comes along straight away, and at other times you have to meet several people before finding someone you're happy to spend months, or even years, talking to regularly about your concerns.

There are several therapeutic modalities to be mindful of:

Person-centred therapy This form of therapy is focused on the clients' experience of themselves rather than the therapist being the expert who interprets and tells people what to do. The therapy is focused on the relationship between the therapist and the client, where the foundation is based on the therapist extending the 'core conditions' to the client, as defined by Carl Rogers. The core conditions are empathy (the therapist trying to understand the client's point of view), congruence (the therapist being a genuine person) and unconditional positive regard (the therapist being non-judgemental). This is a non-directive approach, where the client or patient, rather than the therapist, is encouraged to lead the sessions.

Existential/humanistic therapy Existential therapy focuses on the anxiety that occurs when someone confronts the conflicts that are present in life. These could be questions around identity, purpose, meaning, death, isolation and freedom. If you want to examine the big questions in your life, this is the place to do it.

Psychodynamic therapy This is based on Freud's original principles of bringing the unconscious mind into consciousness, which involves helping people to experience, understand and interpret their thoughts and emotions in order to resolve them. This approach takes the view that our unconscious holds on to painful feelings and memories, which are too difficult for the conscious mind to process. This is a much more directive approach, where the therapist may guide the session at times.

Cognitive behavioural therapy CBT is extremely popular due to its structured nature and is often what is offered on the NHS for exactly this reason. CBT aims to change your thoughts to change your behaviour. It is heavily directive and practical, with homework tasks often given between sessions. There are great benefits of CBT when cognition and patterns of thinking are unhelpful, such as in perfectionism or anxiety. If your primary concerns are emotional, however, you might find something lacking here. I often meet with people who have tried CBT for eating disorders and found that although it helps somewhat, they feel that something is missing and they are at greater risk of relapse. In my experience (and I've trained in CBT-E, which is CBT for eating disorders), an emotional component is needed on top of the cognitive and behavioural in order to effectively remove an eating disorder from a person's brain.

Emotion-focused therapy This approach views emotions as being essential in helping individuals to understand the world and to respond effectively to various demands, challenges and situations. This approach focuses on emotions, as the name suggests, and posits that people are more likely to develop emotional difficulties in adulthood if their childhood experiences involve being raised in an environment that models emotions as being unacceptable or overwhelming. The goal is to help people become more aware of their emotions and be able to express them more constructively.

Acceptance and commitment therapy The objective of ACT is not elimination of difficult feelings; instead it's about learning to be present with whatever life throws at us, including difficult emotions, and to aim to engage in behaviours that are helpful. This approach is, in many ways, the antithesis of CBT, as there is no challenging of thoughts or beliefs. The principles are acceptance, values, being in the present moment, cognitive defusion, psychological flexibility and committed action. This is a heavily directive approach with many practical tools.

Eye movement desensitisation and reprogramming EMDR is a strange little therapy that primarily works by following the therapist's finger from left to right, just moving your eyes, in similar patterns as happens during REM (rapid eye movement) sleep. It sounds bizarre, and yet it is continuously being shown to be highly effective in processing trauma, particularly trauma arising from a single event, such as an assault or a natural disaster. When it comes to single-event trauma, it's often more effective than regular talking therapy.

Integrative therapy combines several modalities and applies those that work for each individual person or concern. This is the approach many therapists now take, and which I myself have adopted. I have a person-centred foundation, with additional training in CBT, ACT and existential therapy, with a dash of psychodynamic principles here and there where appropriate.

Nutrition counselling A nutrition counsellor is a nutrition professional, usually registered with the Association for Nutrition (in the UK), or HCPC if they're a dietitian, who has some psychological training and works with disordered eating and body-image concerns. This label has also become more popular among practitioners who work primarily within a non-diet and Health At Every Size © framework, using principles of intuitive eating rather than a traditional weight-focused approach. Because of this, if your concerns have strong psychological and emotional components, it's worth double-checking that the practitioner you want to work with has some basic therapeutic training.

Where to find therapy/counselling?

Unfortunately, therapy is not as accessible worldwide as I would like it to be. It can be expensive, or there can be long waiting lists and hoops to jump through to access free or low-cost therapy. Depending on where you are located in the world, you may be able to access therapy via a national health service provider, charities and not-for-profit organisations in your area, school or university student services, counselling directories, searching a professional register (in the UK this could be the BPS, BACP or UKCP registers), or through private/work insurance policies.

For some services, you may be required to have a diagnosis to be referred on. This is something you can discuss with your primary care provider or general practitioner. If you are self-referring to private therapy services, a diagnosis will likely not be required.

Questions to ask a potential therapist or nutrition counsellor

- What is your experience in working with food and body issues?
- Will you tell me what to eat? (The answer for a therapist should absolutely be NO.)
- Do you have any training in food and body issues?
- Do you operate within a weight-centric or weight-inclusive paradigm? (The answer should be the latter.)
- Are you aware of the impacts of weight stigma and diet culture?

When you find the right therapist or nutrition counsellor, and you are ready to commit to the work, it can be life changing. It is never too late to start and, yes, your concerns are absolutely valid. The longest relationship you have is with yourself and your body, and if you want to take this step to work on that, more power to you.

Resources and Further Reading

Counselling and therapy directories

https://www.bacp.co.uk/search/Register
https://www.bacp.co.uk/search/Therapists
https://www.bps.org.uk/find-psychologist
https://www.counselling-directory.org.uk/

Worksheets

For full-page pdf versions of worksheets in this book please go to:

https://www.pixieturnernutrition.com/resources

Further reading

The Joy of Being Selfish, Michelle Elman
Is Butter a Carb?, Rosie Saunt and Helen West
Intuitive Eating, Evelyn Tribole and Elyse Resch
Eat Up!, Ruby Tandoh
How to Build a Healthy Brain, Kimberley Wilson

Emotional Agility, Susan David
Happy Fat, Sofie Hagen
Hunger, Roxane Gay
When Food is Love, Geneen Roth
The No Need to Diet Book, Pixie Turner

Acknowledgements

It's time for me to say thank you to a wonderful bunch of people!

To the entire team that has made this book possible, who believed in it, and believed in me.

To my incredible colleague Hebe who works with me and read through the entire manuscript for me.

To the cohort of students who studied counselling and psychotherapy alongside me. I will never forget the blood, sweat and many, many tears we endured to survive that training.

To my wonderful family and friends who I value so much in my life.

To every client who has contacted me, trusted me, opened up to me and shared with me. You are my greatest teachers.

Finally, to the great love of my life, my cat Mimi, who was always there for cuddles through power writing and writer's block alike.

References

1 Sadalla, E. and Burroughs, J. (1981), 'Profiles in Eating: Sexy vegetarians and other diet-based social stereotypes. *Psychology Today*, 15(10), p.51

2 Bongers, P. and Jansen, A. (2016), 'Emotional eating is not what you think it is and emotional eating scales do not measure what you think they measure', *Frontiers in Psychology*, 7, p.1932

3 Brownell, K.D. and Rodin, J. (1994), 'Medical, metabolic, and psychological effects of weight cycling', *Archives of Internal Medicine*, 154(12), pp1325–30

4 Puhl, R.M., Lessard, L.M., et al. (2021), 'The roles of experienced and internalized weight stigma in healthcare experiences: Perspectives of adults engaged in weight management across six countries', *PloS One*, 16(6), p.e0251566

5 Vanderbilt, D., Young, R., et al. (2008), 'Asthma severity and PTSD symptoms among inner city children: A pilot study', *Journal of Trauma & Dissociation*, 9(2), pp191–207

6 Nummenmaa, L., Glerean, E., et al. (2014), 'Bodily maps of emotions', *Proceedings of the National Academy of Sciences*, 111(2), pp646–51

7 Mason, S.M., Flint, A. J., et al. (2013), 'Abuse victimization in childhood or adolescence and risk of food addiction in adult women', *Obesity*, 21(12), ppE775–81

8 Breland, J.Y., Donalson, R., et al. (2018), 'Trauma exposure and disordered eating: A qualitative study', *Women & Health*, 58(2), pp160–74

9 Mackay, P.S.E. (2014), 'Psychological determinants of emotional eating: The role of attachment, psychopathological symptom distress, love attitudes and perceived hunger', *Current Research in Psychology*, 5(2), pp77–88

10 https://publications.parliament.uk/pa/cm5801/cmselect/ cmwomeq/805/80502.htm

11 Davis-Coelho, K., Waltz, J. and Davis-Coelho, B. (2000), 'Awareness and prevention of bias against fat clients in psychotherapy', *Professional Psychology: Research and Practice*, 31(6), pp682–4

12 Swift, J.A., Hanlon, S., et al. (2013), 'Weight bias among UK trainee dietitians, doctors, nurses and nutritionists', *Journal of Human Nutrition and Dietetics*, 26(4), pp395–402

13 Flegal, K.M., Kit, B.K., et al. (2013), 'Association of all-cause mortality with overweight and obesity using standard body mass index categories', *JAMA*, 309(1), p.71

14 Bacon L. and Aphramor L. (2011), 'Weight science: Evaluating the evidence for a paradigm shift', *Nutrition Journal*, 10(1), pp1–13

15 NIH Technology Assessment Conference Panel (1992), 'Methods for voluntary weight loss and control', *Annals of Internal Medicine*, 116(11), pp942–9

16 French, S.A., Jeffery, R.W. and Forster, J.L. (1994), 'Dieting status and its relationship to weight, dietary intake, and physical activity changes over two years in a working population', *Obesity Research and Clinical Practice*, 2(2), pp135–44

17 https://www.ipsos.com/en/global-weight-and-actions

18 https://www.mintel.com/press-centre/food-and-drink/brits-lose-count-of-their-calories-over-a-third-of-brits-dont-know-how-many-calories-they-consume-on-a-typical-day

19 Müller, M.J., Bosy-Westphal, A. and Heymsfield, S.B. (2010), 'Is there evidence for a set point that regulates human body weight?' *F1000 Medicine Reports*, 2:59,

20 Jiang, K. (2021) June, 'Review on binge eating disorder: Theories, influencing factors and treatments', in *2021 2nd International Conference on Mental Health and Humanities Education (ICMHHE 2021)*, pp586–90, Atlantis Press

21 Fisher, J.O. and Birch, L.L. (1999), 'Restricting access to palatable foods affects children's behavioral response, food selection, and intake', *American Journal of Clinical Nutrition*, 69(6), pp1264–72

22 Neumark-Sztainer, D., Bauer, K.W., et al. (2010), 'Family weight talk and dieting: How much do they matter for body dissatisfaction and disordered eating behaviors in adolescent girls?', *Journal of Adolescent Health*, 47(3), pp270–6

23 Puhl, R. and Suh, Y. (2015), 'Stigma and eating and weight disorders', *Current Psychiatry* Reports, 17(3), p.10

24 Bayer, V., Robert-McComb, J.J., et al. (2017), 'Investigating the influence of shame, depression, and distress tolerance on the relationship between internalized homophobia and binge eating in lesbian and bisexual women', *Eating Behaviors*, 24, pp39–44

25 Freud, A. (1937), *The Ego and the Mechanisms of Defense*, London: Hogarth Press and Institute of Psycho-Analysis

26 Polivy, J. and Pliner, P. (2015), "She got more than me": Social comparison and the social context of eating', *Appetite*, 86, pp88–95

27 Fitzsimmons-Craft, E.E. (2017), 'Eating disorder-related social comparison in college women's everyday lives', *International Journal of Eating Disorders*, 50(8), pp893–905

28 Brewer, R., Cook, R. and Bird, G. (2016), 'Alexithymia: A general deficit of interoception', *Royal Society Open Science*, 3(10), p.150664

29 Mattila, A.K., Saarni, S.I., et al. (2009), 'Alexithymia and health-related quality of life in a general population', *Psychosomatics*, 50(1), pp59–68

30 Shank, L.M., Tanofsky-Kraff, M., et al. (2019). 'The association between alexithymia and eating behavior in children and adolescents', *Appetite*, 142, p.104381

31 Curran, T. and Hill, A.P. (2019), 'Perfectionism is increasing over time: A meta-analysis of birth cohort differences from 1989 to 2016', *Psychological Bulletin*, 145(4), p.410

32 Nilsson, K., Sundbom, E. and Hägglöf, B. (2008), 'A longitudinal study of perfectionism in adolescent onset anorexia nervosa-restricting type', *European Eating Disorders Review: The Professional Journal of the Eating Disorders Association*, 16(5), pp386–94

33 Wang, H. and Li, J. (2017), 'Positive perfectionism, negative perfectionism, and emotional eating: The mediating role of stress', *Eating Behaviors*, 26, pp45–9

34 Lehto, R. and Stein, K. (2009), 'Death anxiety: An analysis of an evolving concept', *Research and Theory for Nursing Practice*, 23(1), pp23–41

35 https://www.theatlantic.com/health/archive/2017/02/eating-toward-immortality/515658/

36 Nummenmaa, L., Glerean, E., et al. (2014), 'Bodily maps of emotions', *Proceedings of the National Academy of Sciences*, 111(2), pp646–51

Index

Note: page numbers in *italics* refer to information contained in tables.